The Politics of Medicine in China

Other Titles in This Series

Westview Special Studies
on China and East Asia

*The Politics of Medicine in China:
The Policy Process, 1949-1977*

David M. Lampton

David Lampton describes the preliberation health
system in China and how preliberation experiences
and postliberation problems have shaped health policy
in the PRC. Drawing on a vast range of primary materials including interviews, local Chinese-language
newspapers, and travel reports, he explains the
reasons for health policy change in the PRC and draws
more general conclusions about Chinese politics and
change.

This study concentrates on medical education, research, financing, health care delivery, traditional
medicine, professional life, and mass campaigns. Dr.
Lampton summarizes his findings in five areas: (1) the
Chinese have made substantial progress in health
work, which reflects the unique blending of prerevo-
lution legacies and postliberation aspirations and
programs. (2) At all times, health policy has reflected economic constraints, organizational and
elite conflict, and the response of the Chinese populace. (3) Rather than one unified policy process in
China during the last twenty-eight years, the very
structure of the policy process has changed in response to economic and policy difficulties. (4) There
has been a tendency for policy-making authority to
gravitate toward the medical bureaucracy, despite re-
peated attempts to diminish that role. (5) Finally,
there has been a continual effort to expand the number of social sectors with a direct impact on the
health bureaucracy. Whether or not peasant interests
have, in fact, been institutionalized is one of the
major questions to be answered in the post-Mao era.

David Lampton received his doctorate in political
science from Stanford University and is now assistant
professor of political science at the Ohio State University, where he is affiliated with the Mershon
Center.

The Politics of Medicine in China

The Policy Process, 1949-1977

David M. Lampton

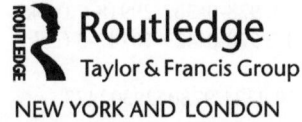

Routledge
Taylor & Francis Group

NEW YORK AND LONDON

First published in paperback 2024

First published 1977 by Westview Press

Published 2019 by Routledge
605 Third Avenue, New York, NY 10158

and by Routledge
4 Park Square, Milton Park, Abingdon, Oxon OX14 4RN

Routledge is an imprint of the Taylor & Francis Group, an informa business

Copyright © 1977, 2019, 2024 Taylor & Francis

Library of Congress Cataloging in Publication Data

Lampton, David M.
    The politics of medicine in China.

    (Westview special studies on China and East
Asia)
    Bibliography: p.
    1. Medical policy--China. 2. China--Politics
and government--1949-   I. Title.
RA395.C53L36   362.1'0951   77-8291

Publisher's Note
The publisher has gone to great lengths to ensure the quality of this reprint but points out that some imperfections in the original copies may be apparent.

ISBN 13: 978-0-367-28372-8 (hbk)
ISBN 13: 978-0-367-29918-7 (pbk)
ISBN 13: 978-0-429-30247-3 (ebk)

DOI: 10.4324/9780429302473

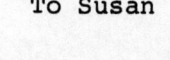
To Susan

In the daytime few are in the
     fields.

At night ghosts sing under the
     moon.

When shall we see the end of our
     suffering?

And when shall happiness touch
     us?

                    Traditional peasant lament

CONTENTS

PART 4

THE CULTURAL REVOLUTION:
COALITION POLITICS

LIST OF TABLES AND FIGURES

ACKNOWLEDGMENTS

Ever since beginning this enterprise, I have been the recipient of large doses of encouragement from my wife Susan, to whom this book is dedicated, and my two families. In conducting my research and thinking about health politics in China, I have mined the intellectual resources of scores of individuals, only a few of whom I can presently thank. John Wilson Lewis has been a teacher proficient in both the arts of listening and criticizing; for both his skills I am thankful. Michel Oksenberg has contributed enormously to my understanding of the Chinese policy process and has repeatedly made resources available which improved my work and permitted me to expeditiously get on with the job. I have been Gabriel Almond's student since my undergraduate years, and if this study has succeeded in achieving a comparative perspective, it is in no small part due to his influence. It is often difficult for an "area specialist" to tap the accumulated expertise of another profession, but Dr. Paul Basch of the Stanford School of Medicine made my task easier by introducing me to the international health literature. Finally, I would like to thank Thomas P. Bernstein, Stephen Goldstein, Harry Harding, Peter N. Lee, Victor Li, Robert North, and Seiichiro Takagi for commenting on this research at one point or another.

In addition to those individuals mentioned above, I would like to thank Ezra Vogel for making his extensive interview protocols available. Similarly, Susan B. Rifkin was of great help and encouragement to me in Hong Kong. She read an earlier draft of the entire manuscript and made available her interviews with traditional Chinese physicians.

Those I interviewed in Hong Kong were my mentors as well. I will not mention their names only because I know that most would prefer to remain anonymous. I hope to retain their friendship throughout the years. Of special importance are two wonderful women in Hong Kong: One showed my

xv

wife and me great affection and helped my work
immeasurably. The other's veritable thirst for
traditional medicines brought the entire rainbow of
Chinese drugs right into our living room.

While in Hong Kong in 1972 and 1973, I profited
from the services provided by the Universities Service Centre, its attentive and efficient staff, its
able director, B. Michael Frolic, and its assistant
director, John Dolfin. Upon my return to the United
States, I was fortunate enough to be able to spend
the 1973-1974 academic year at the University of
Michigan's Center for Chinese Studies. Both Albert
Feuerwerker and Rhoads Murphey made that a most
productive period for me. Finally, my colleagues
and the staff at The Ohio State University have
been most supportive. I especially appreciate Ms.
Connie Gaib's typing and the editorial assistance
of Mervyn W. Adams Seldon.

The financial support of several institutions
has made the research and production of this volume
possible. The United States Office of Education
awarded me a Fulbright-Hays Grant for the 1972-1973
period. The Mabelle McLeod Lewis Memorial Fund
provided me with essential write-up money. Finally,
the Josiah Macy, Jr. Foundation made my stay at
Michigan possible. To all these organizations I say
thanks. With all this help, the least I can do is
assume full responsibility for the results.

INTRODUCTION

Today, medical analysts and officials concerned with the United States and the Third World are searching for alternative means by which to bring needed health services to their people.[1] For a mixture of reasons, including China's visible success, cultural resonance, and historical accident, the Chinese health experience has come to occupy an exalted place among the many possible alternatives. In the process of assessing the applicability of China's medical programs, however, insufficient attention has been directed toward analyzing the concrete results of past policies and the reasons for subsequent policy change. While this volume is specifically concerned with analyzing the reasons for policy change, and deriving a coherent view of the Chinese political process from that analysis, this discussion should provide the background for informed public policy debate here and abroad.

This study has the objective of examining and explaining changes in Chinese health care policy during the 1949-1977 period. The questions which this study seeks to answer are: why have policies changed, why have they moved in the directions they have, and what does all this tell us about the Chinese policy process? Seven important areas of medical policy will be considered: medical education, medical research, the structure of the health care delivery system, service financing, the conditions of physician employment, traditional medicine, and mass campaigns.*

---

*A comprehensive study of medical issues with political significance would include an analysis of policies in the areas of birth control, food inspection, industrial safety, environmental health, and pharmaceutical production.

Every polity has, and needs, several levels of
policy in order to meet the needs of the present
and provide the flexibility with which to deal with
the future. It is necessary to specify what kind of
policy is of concern here. The distinction between
two types of policy is particularly useful in the
Chinese case: (a) normative policy and (b) action
policy.

Normative health policy can best be understood
as a set of long-term goals and values supporting
more short-term programs. Its links with concrete
endeavors are indirect because normative policy does
not provide precise guidance to those involved in
implementation. China's normative health policy has
not changed significantly from the formula enunciated at the First National Health Conference of
August 1950.[2] Its four enduring dimensions have
been: (1) Emphasis on preventive medicine. (2) Promotion of the union of traditional and western medicine. (3) Provision of health services for "the
broad masses." (4) Utilization of mass health campaigns and mobilization of the people to solve their
own health problems. Changes in these four broad
principles have been negligible.

Action policy, in contrast, seeks to take general guidelines and translate them into concrete programs. This involves the planning function. Because political and economic resources are scarce,
any normative policy inevitably embodies aspirations
which cannot all be met simultaneously. Consequently, the health policy-making leadership has always
had to make choices and set priorities. Similarly,
because human and material resources are limited,
target groups have had to be identified (to the
exclusion of other sectors of the society) and an
all-inclusive word like "the masses" has not been
of much help in this task. For instance, if the
criterion for distribution is "efficiency," or "curative services for the greatest number," this creates
an urban bias which is objectionable if "equity" is
the yardstick by which alternatives are evaluated.
If, on the other hand, the guide for distribution
is "put the stress on rural areas," is maximum use
being made of scarce manpower and medical resources?
What happens to the quality of care available to
urbanites?

Action policy, in short, deals with a broad
range of issues: the construction and location of
medical institutions, health financing, medical
education, distribution of services, types of research to be promoted or tolerated, and guidelines

for professional life. The relationship between
normative and action policy is dynamic, with the
former setting direction and the latter establishing
concrete priorities and modes of implementation. In
the absence of universal value agreement, however,
making action policy is frequently a conflict laden
process. Identifying those characteristics of the
Chinese policy process which most nearly account for
the shape of, and changes in, action policy is the
objective of this study.

THE FRAMEWORK FOR ANALYSIS

Three variables are important in understanding
the generation of policy in any system; these factors seem particularly salient in the Chinese case.
First, who have been the persons formally charged
with responsibility for making health care action
policy and how has the composition of this elite
changed? Secondly, having identified the salient
leadership, what have been "its" perceptions of the
problems?[3] More accurately, has the leadership been
divided over differing perceptions and have these
cleavages had important political consequences?
Thirdly, given a knowledge of leadership composition
and leadership perceptions, what political and
economic resources have been available to these persons to achieve their predispositions? What social
resistances have leaders anticipated (or encountered)
in pursuing any given policy line? What strategies
have different participants devised in order to
overcome these cleavages and resistances?
While the above variables are central to understanding policy outcomes, these factors interact in
a context; that context is a network of organizations, political arenas, or policy-making forums.[4]
These policy-making structures condition the perceptions of leaders and make available only certain
categories of political and material resources. The
structure of the policy-making system constricts
the flow of information, determines the level at
which specific decisions are made, and dictates
recruitment patterns. Health politics, then, involves two broad areas of political conflict: (1)
What kind of policy structure is "best" and, (2)
within the agreed upon structure, what should the
specific content of action policies be?
Major decisions relating to the structure of
the policy-making system are always made at the
Central Committee and Politburo levels. Structural

alterations were made in 1955-1958, 1960, and 1967-1969. Each of these structural changes marked the beginning of a new policy era.

Explaining change in political structures and public policies has been an enduring concern of political science; it is certainly the raison d'être for this study. Changes in policy-making structure have resulted from the fact that every mechanism for making public decisions alienates certain sectors of the leadership and society and generates policies with identifiable economic and administrative defects. These defects and divisions have created pressures for changes in the policy-making mechanism itself. As we shall see in the chapters to follow, and analyze in detail in the final chapter, these pressures have given rise to three distinct patterns of health policy-making in China during the last twenty-eight years. Every change in the decision-making system has brought different mixes of leadership, perceptions, resources, and constraints in its wake. Medical policy has reflected those alterations.

The behavioral tradition, as important as it has been in raising consciousness concerning the structural reasons for man's political behavior, has down-played the importance of leadership. Plato, Machiavelli, Hobbes, Mosca, Pareto, Lenin, and Mao (each in his own way to be sure) have all emphasized the paramount role of the political leader and the malleability of the social environment. To these political theorists and practitioners, as to Henry David Thoreau, the clay of the earth is soft and impressionable under the feet of man. Our analytic perspective will straddle the leadership and behavioral traditions. It recognizes that policy-makers are crucial and that their goals and strategies are important; it is also cognizant that a leader's perceptions and options are severely influenced and constrained by his background, the organizational context in which he is embedded, the social pressures to which he is subjected, and the pervasive scarcity of material and political resources.

PROBLEMS OF DATA AND INFERENCE

It is customary for analysts of China to lie prostrate at the temple of uncertainty, to make incantations about perseverance in the face of adversity, and to engage in a ritual confessional about methodological inadequacies. In fact, the

trail of the pious is so well worn that I will only
mention a few of the problems which were, and are,
particularly nettlesome.

The major information problem concerns not its
quantity (which is overwhelming), but its quality.
By quality I mean, how precise a statement will the
data unambiguously support? "Low quality" information is that which, for example, says that "health
expenditures rose 500 percent in the last decade."
Data of "good quality" would say, in contrast, that
"health expenditures, in curative facilities at the
county and above levels, rose 5 percent in the
first quarter of 1965 due to several factors." This
kind of information is usually unavailable. When
"good" data are located, they usually cover short
periods and pertain to atypical examples.

Secondly, the analytic framework outlined above
would profit from substantial background data on
political leaders and information relating to leadership interaction in decision-making organs. This
kind of information is very rare; when such data are
released (e.g., 1955, 1959, 1967, and 1976), it is
usually in the context of a major leadership shakeup
in which information is used as a weapon with which
to club political opponents. Because of the use to
which such information is put, one has to treat it
gingerly.

Because information emanating from the Chinese
political system is generally either of low specifi-
city (or so specific that one is unable to general-
ize from it) and/or of low reliability, the author
sought to corroborate and supplement official
reports by unofficial appraisals. Because extensive
field research has not been possible, one is forced
to rely upon refugee interviews and/or Taiwan sources. In gathering data for this study, I used
refugee interviews (those conducted by myself and
others) and rarely used Taiwan sources. There are
two reasons for not relying heavily on Taiwanese
information: First, Taipei apparently has not
devoted much attention to examining China's health
and social welfare system. Taiwan either does not
have, or has not released, information which is not
readily available in the public, non-Taiwanese,
domain. Secondly, the invaluable documents which
have come to us through Taiwan, such as the Lien-
chiang papers,[5] just add detail to a general picture
which had already emerged from the communist press,
the variable stream of visitors to China, and
refugees from the mainland. In short, there was
little need to rely on Taipei's information. Had I

been studying the militia in Fukien Province, Taiwanese sources might have proved crucial.

The problem of interview reliability is a more knotty issue and one that can only be recognized. Nothing can be done to eliminate the biases of proud persons who have strong feelings about a homeland they felt compelled to leave. Nevertheless, refugee interviews are the only even reasonable supplements and correctives to the controlled Chinese media. Perhaps the major utility of interviews is as a supplement to data culled from the mass media. For instance, Chinese news sources have talked for years about financial difficulties in hospitals, but it remained for interviewees to describe how great the problems were and what the responses had been. Similarly, knowledge of informal lines of authority is critical to understanding the actual lines of decision-making power in medical institutions. Interviews are the only substitute for personal participant-observer status.

The most dangerous biases which interviewees inject into a scholarly analysis are not immediately obvious. The overt hostility toward the People's Republic on the part of some interviewees was apparent and could be minimized by asking questions which elicited quantitative responses. The real danger, however, is that the interviewer will unwittingly adopt the factional (or clique) model of Chinese politics without carefully assessing alternative explanations. The people I interviewed rarely sought the explanation for political behavior in divergent interests which resulted from impersonal social structures and roles. They generally believed that political behavior derived from personal relationships and cliques among leaders.* Those individuals interviewed spoke of Chinese politics in terms rather reminiscent of the Ch'ing court with eunuchs conspiring against one another for the ear of the Empress Dowager. This view is not inconsistent with the 1976 purge of Chiang Ch'ing. While

---

*A fact which is often overlooked is that personal relationships are important in all political settings. There has been a tendency to seek the explanation for Chinese political behavior in factions alone, rather than seeing personal relationships as one resource, among many, that must be utilized by the successful policy-maker.

personal (family, loyalty, lineage, and friendship) relationships may be more salient in the Chinese context than in other cultural settings, introducing a structural component to the explanation helps us understand why certain lines of cleavage have persisted, irrespective of the personalities involved.

In sum, the issue of the biases of Chinese refugees brings us to a restatement of the purpose of this study. It is an attempt to acknowledge the obvious centrality of leaders to policy outcomes and, at the same time, to specify the constraints placed upon those individuals by the structures in which they operate and by the society stretching in an endless expanse beyond the government's doors. Only when we have an understanding of how health policy was produced in China, and of the reasons why it was changed, can we assess the applicability and the desirability of adopting that experience elsewhere.

NOTES

1. Victor W. Sidel and Ruth Sidel, Serve the People (New York: Josiah Macy, Jr. Foundation, 1973); also, Susan Rifkin, "Public Health in China: Is the Experience Relevant to Other Less Developed Nations?", Social Science and Medicine 7 (1973):249-257.

2. For a contemporary Chinese report on the First National Health Conference see, "The Correct Direction in People's Health Work," Hsin-hua Yueh-pao [New China monthly] 13 (1950):166.

3. Alexander George, "The 'Operational Code': A Neglected Approach to the Study of Political Leaders and Decision-Making," International Studies Quarterly 13, no. 2 (1969):190-222.

4. David M. Lampton, "Policy Arenas and the Study of Chinese Politics," Studies in Comparative Communism 7, no. 4 (1974):409-413; see also, Michel Oksenberg, "The Chinese Policy Process and the Public Health Issue: An Arena Approach," Studies in Comparative Communism 7, no. 4 (1974):375-408.

5. C. S. Chen and Charles Ridley, Rural People's Communes in Lien-chiang (Stanford: Hoover Institution Press, 1969).

PART 1

PRE-REVOLUTIONARY LEGACIES AND POST-REVOLUTIONARY CHANGE

Chapter 1
THE PRE-LIBERATION MEDICAL SYSTEM AND POST-REVOLUTIONARY CHANGE

INTRODUCTION

Analysts of the People's Republic of China sometimes are like biblical historians, designating all before the "creation" as "chaos." In reality, however, post-revolutionary change has proceeded from the accumulated experiences and resources of Chinese traditional diagnostic and therapeutic practices, western-style medicine, and the revolutionary health system built by the Red Army in the 1930s and 1940s. While the purpose of this book is to identify and explain change in medical policy throughout the post-1949 period, two contexts must be provided: First, what were the characteristics of the pre-liberation Chinese "medical system," what changes were already occurring, and what was the state of health of the Chinese people at liberation? Secondly, what identifiable impact have post-1949 health policies had on the physical wellbeing of the Chinese people?

THE TRADITIONAL CHINESE FOUNDATION IN HEALTH CARE

The seminal work on the theory and techniques of traditional Chinese medicine (Chung-i) is the Yellow Emperor's Classic of Internal Medicine (Huang Ti Nei Ching Su Wen) which is of uncertain age and origin.[1] The Nei Ching was written in the form of a dialogue between the legendary Yellow Emperor (2697-2597 B.C.) and his court physician, Ch'i Po. In the course of their extended conversation the doctor explained the origins of, and cures for, disease. The keystone of the Chinese medical tradition is the notion that medicine is the art of maintaining health, not curing disease. Chairman Mao Tse-tung's subsequent emphasis on preventive medicine is perfectly consistent with this legacy.

3

The key to maintaining health, the Nei Ching argued, was the maintenance of a balance between the universal forces of yin and yang. Once the balance between yin and yang had been disrupted, a complex diagnostic process had to be initiated. In order to define the nature of the imbalance affecting the body, the concordances between yin and yang, the seasons, particular body organs, specific foods, and individual mental states had to be known. Diagnosis, according to the Nei Ching, could be accomplished by using several methods: carefully examining the patient's six pulses, observing the patient's appearance, and, occasionally, analyzing the individual's dreams. Once the source of the bodily imbalance had been determined, a course of treatment could be prescribed. The correct use of indigenous herbs and other pharmaceutical agents was considered essential.

The treatment most well-known in the West is acupuncture. It, too, was first mentioned in the Nei Ching, although Veith says that its use must well antedate the book itself. Acupuncture was a way of stimulating, or maintaining, what we would call a "dynamic equilibrium" between the yin and the yang. It was believed that the cosmic forces of the yin and yang flowed through the body's twelve "meridians" and that disease frequently was a result of the obstruction of these channels. By inserting needles at specified points such obstructions could supposedly be removed and the normal circulation of forces restored.[2]

These concepts of health, physiology, diagnosis, and treatment are the foundation upon which later traditional medical practice was built. Using the concepts of the Nei Ching, obstetrics and gynecology became identifiable specialties as early as 85 B.C. Ch'un Yu-i, a famous Han physician, used drugs to induce labor. In addition, the abortion inducing properties of certain naturally occurring drugs were known and employed.[3] These same agents are now being systematically analyzed and used by various research facilities in the People's Republic of China. Concurrent with this interest in obstetrics and gynecology, the specialty of pediatrics appeared. In 26 B.C., Li Chu-kuo published a nineteen volume work on the diseases of women and children.

At the same time that interest was being demonstrated in the above specialties, Shen-nung, a famous pharmacist of the early Han Dynasty (206 B.C.- 222 A.D.), was compiling China's first pharmacopoeia, the Classic on Local Herbs (Pen-ts'ao Ching).[4]

4

During successive generations, the catalogue of
Chinese herbs grew, reaching its pinnacle in the
work of the famous Ming druggist Li Shih-chen.
Referring to Li and several of his contemporaries,
Lee T'ao says,

> They made intensive studies into the principles
> of pathology and drug therapy, while doing much
> to combat mysticism and superstition, including
> the concept that the main aim of medicine was
> to prolong life by miraculous means.[5]

Not only did gynecology, obstetrics, pediatrics,
and pharmacology have rather early beginnings in
China, so did surgery, under the skillful leadership of Hua T'o.[6] According to the Book of the
Later Han (Hou-han Shu), Hua performed major
abdominal and orthopedic operations. The surgical
tradition in China, after Hua, remained dormant
until the Yuan Dynasty (1234-1368 A.D.).

> The Mongols in their conquests depended chiefly
> on their cavalry and their horsemen suffered
> frequently from bone fractures and dislocations
> of joints. Hence great attention was paid to
> surgery and orthopedics.[7]

This latent surgical tradition was subsequently
promoted during the Ch'ing Dynasty (1644-1911 A.D.)
by the Emperor K'ang Hsi, who had a personal interest
in dissection. The emperor ordered that prisoners
condemned to death be used for medical purposes.
Despite these infrequent flirtations with surgery,
Chinese generally resisted the idea of physicians
cutting the skin because defacement of the body was
considered an unfilial act.[8] Probably more importantly, the death rate for those who underwent
surgery was undoubtedly appalling.

Quite early, the Chinese became interested in
the maintenance of ethical and professional standards in the practice of medicine. As Croizier
notes, the Rites of the Chou Dynasty (Chou-li)
acknowledged the state's responsibility for control-
ling medical practice by administering qualifying
examinations to prospective practitioners.[9] Whether
or not this system, in fact, had any impact will
never be known. Subsequently, both the Sung Dynasty
(907-1279 A.D.) and the Yuan Dynasty (1234-1368 A.D.)
placed controls on medical practitioners. Departments of Medical Education were established in all
provinces for the purpose of

. . . examining physicians and medical personnel holding official posts, censoring
published medical books, identifying medicinal
herbs, training medical students and directing
medical work generally.[10]

Looking at the record as a whole, traditional
Chinese medicine was to bequeath three important
legacies to the post-1949 regime: First, it was
widely accepted by the people and it represented an
integrated world view in which daily activities had
to be structured in such a way as to maintain health.
The communist emphasis on prevention is entirely
consistent with this tradition. Secondly, from an
early time it had been accepted that the state had
the responsibility to regulate medical practice in
the social interest. While such a responsibility
was observed more in the breach than the fact, the
communists could easily build upon this expectation
in constructing a system of state medical care.
Finally, Chung-i had emphasized the therapeutic
value of locally obtained plant and animal materials;
this represented a substantial resource, considering
the weakness of the modern pharmaceutical industry
in the post-liberation period.
In 1954, Chairman Mao was paraphrased as having
said,

. . . traditional Chinese medicine has a history of several thousand years. . . . Even up
to the present, still upwards of five hundred
million people in the country rely on traditional Chinese medicine for treatment of their
diseases. . . . For this reason, . . . the
contribution made by traditional Chinese
medicine is immense indeed, while that of
western medicine is insignificant in comparison.[11]

THE LEGACY OF WESTERN MEDICINE PRIOR TO 1949

With the arrival of the Portuguese in Macao in
1504 A.D., western medicine gained its first foot-
hold in China. During the next three centuries,
western practitioners occasionally landed in China
as part of a ship's crew. Despite the fact that
by the early 1800s smallpox vaccinations were
periodically administered by these individuals, the
impact of western medicine was not great. This
reflected the fact that European medical practices

6

were not necessarily more advanced than those of the
Chinese. Equally important, the imperial Chinese
authorities perceived the westerners to constitute
more of a threat than the diseases they claimed to
be able to cure.

The extensive penetration of China by western-
style medicine had to await the opening of China
with the Bible and the battering ram, the latter
being the most important. While three medical
missionaries (John Livingstone, Peter Parker,[12] and
Robert Morrison) had established clinics in Macao
and Canton during the first three decades of the
1800s, the extensive diffusion of western medicine
had proven impossible until the opening of China by
the 1842 Treaty of Nanking and the subsequent Treaty
of Tientsin (1858). As a consequence of these two
documents (especially the latter), all China was
opened to medical missionary work. Rapidly, a
symbiotic relationship developed between religion
and medicine. The missionary movement provided
medicine with a vehicle by which it could move into
China and medicine gave the missionaries something
the Chinese needed which they could provide. W. H.
Medhurst graphically described this relationship.

> Though the law which excludes the preacher
> operates equally against the practitioner, yet
> the incipient departure from the letter of the
> enactment may be more likely to take place in
> the case of the dispenser of health than the
> reformer of morals; simply because the Chinese
> feel their need in the one case and not in the
> other.[13]

Because the relationship between medicine and
missionary work was so intimate, nationalistic
Chinese were, and continue to be, ambivalent about
the role of western physicians and hospitals.
Nowhere has this ambivalence been more apparent than
in the writings of Chairman Mao Tse-tung. In the
same year (1939) that Mao extolled the virtues of
Dr. Norman Bethune, a Canadian surgeon working with
the Chinese communists in the Chin-Cha-Chi Border
Region, the Chairman castigated medical missionaries.[14]

> Furthermore, the imperialist powers have never
> slackened their efforts to poison the minds of
> the Chinese people. This is their policy of
> cultural aggression. And it is carried out
> through missionary work, through establishing

7

hospitals and schools, publishing newspapers
and inducing Chinese students to study abroad.
Their aim is to train intellectuals who will
serve their interests and to dupe the people.[15]

The depth of the hatred which the missionary movement engendered among many Chinese had also been
apparent in the Boxer Rebellion of 1900; missionaries
had been particular targets.

The most renowned of the medical institutions
established by Christians in China was Peking Union
Medical College. In the early 1900s, Dr. Thomas
Cochrane of the London Missionary Society was able
to secure a grant from the Empress Dowager in order
to build a medical school in Peking. The Empress
had been willing to fund such an endeavor because
Cochrane had successfully treated the Empress
Dowager's lady-in-waiting. Subsequently, in 1915,
the China Medical Board, a conduit for the Rocke-
feller Foundation, purchased Cochrane's institution
for $200,000; Peking Union Medical College was born.
One of the major commitments which John D. Rocke-
feller, Jr. undertook upon purchasing the institution was to "select only persons of sound sense and
high character, who were sympathetic with the missionary spirit and motive, who were thoroughly
qualified for their work professionally, and who
would dedicate themselves to medical ministration
in China."[16] During the years to follow, Peking
Union Medical College trained some of China's most
able doctors.

Despite the overwhelming influence which
missionary medical work had, the Chinese were moving
ahead themselves. In 1901, Yuan Shih-k'ai organized
the Pei-yang Medical School; by 1916 twenty-six
similar schools had been established.[17] Equally
important, Dr. Wu Lien-teh established the Northern
Manchurian Plague Prevention Bureau in 1912. Despite the political instability in Peking throughout this period, Dr. Wu was able to nurture his
medical system until it consisted of seven major
hospitals.[18] The activities of Shansi's warlord,
Yen Hsi-shan, were important, as well. Yen, like
many Chinese of the first decades of the 1900s, was
troubled by what the adoption of western medical
practices implied for Chung-i. In order to begin
to work out a viable synthesis between the two
schools, Yen established the Taiyuan Research Society
for the Improvement of Chinese Medicine in 1919.[19]

While leaders such as Yen Hsi-shan were trying
to develop a synthesis between traditional Chinese

8

and western-style medical practices, many other
intellectuals called for the abolition of Chung-i.
This tendency was especially strong among those
students who had studied medicine abroad; luminar-
ies such as Sun Yat-sen, Kuo Mo-jo, and Lu Hsun.
Each man, in his own way, rejected traditional
Chinese medicine. In the case of Sun Yat-sen, "this
early training may well have had a profound influence
on the development of the Kuomintang policy of promoting modern medicine and allowing traditional
practice to wither away through official neglect."[20]
The writer, Lu Hsun, was even less veiled in his
denunciation of Chung-i than Sun. One of Lu's
famous essays, "Medicine" (Yao), is a biting criticism of traditional Chinese medical practices.[21]
Like Lu Hsun, Kuo Mo-jo had little patience with
traditional doctors and, as late as the mid-1940s,
told the Yenan Government that the best thing that
could happen to Chung-i would be its early and merci-
ful demise.[22]

       As a consequence of this intellectual environ-
ment, the initial disposition of the Chinese Communist Party toward traditional medicine was not
entirely favorable. Only the arduous years in the
Kiangsi Soviet and the subsequent period in Yenan
made some of the communists modify their views. As
a result of these early attitudes, there was, and
continues to be, a deep ambivalence toward traditional Chinese medicine. Mao expressed this
ambivalence best when he said in Yenan,

     In the Shensi-Kansu-Ningsia Border Region the
     human and animal mortality rates are both very
     high. . . . In such circumstances, to rely
     solely on modern doctors is no solution. Of
     course, modern doctors have advantages over
     doctors of the old type, but if they do not
     concern themselves with the sufferings of the
     people, do not train doctors for the people,
     do not unite with the thousand and more doctors
     and veterinarians of the old type in the Border
     Region and do not help them to make progress,
     then they will actually be helping the witch
     doctors and showing indifference to the high
     human and animal mortality rates.[23]

       Not only was the evolving intellectual climate
a threat to traditional Chinese medicine, so was the
increasing institutionalization of western medicine.
Between 1921 and 1929, forty-five western-style
medical journals began publication. By 1935, there

were thirty-three medical schools and over 500 hospitals.[24] In addition, once the Nationalist Government in Nanking had been established, it set up a Ministry of Health (1929) which drew its leadership from western-style medical schools, especially Peking Union Medical College.[25]

In 1926, Ting Hsien (a model county in Hopeh Province) became the focus of relatively extensive public health, education, and economic programs.[26] After the Japanese invasion of 1937, the Nationalists announced their intention to build a health system in which every county would have at least one hospital or health center. William Y. Chen claims that by the end of World War II there were some 1,775 county health centers and 26 provincial hospitals. This, however, seems unlikely if for no other reason than the Nationalists did not control that many counties.[27]

Not only was a western-style health infrastructure being built, and an intellectual climate evolving to support it, the medical profession was becoming more organized. The Chinese Medical Association (CMA) had been founded in the second decade of the 1900s and soon became the focus of elite medical activity. The first eight presidents of the CMA were European and American trained physicians who had received their educations at Yale, Cambridge, Pennsylvania, London, Harvard, and Edinburgh.[28] The Association pushed for heightened clinical, research and teaching standards and frequently demanded the licensing of traditional Chinese practitioners. Such attempts were continually resisted by groups of traditional Chinese doctors throughout the 1920s and 1930s.

While we shall momentarily examine the medical care system in the communist base areas during the 1930s and 1940s, the four most important pre-liberation legacies of western-style medicine should be identified: First, the combined efforts of foreign medical missionaries and the Kuomintang resulted in the start of a hospital system and the introduction of public health techniques. Many truly progressive experiments were undertaken, such as the use of paramedics in Ting Hsien. Later communist policies would bear a remarkable resemblance to these early efforts. Secondly, as the western-style medical system grew, it came into increasing conflict with Chung-i; friction is apparent in the 1970s, as well. Thirdly, as western-style medicine became more institutionalized, its practitioners came to occupy ever more important policy-making roles in the

10

national government, roles they were reluctant to
relinquish once the Chinese Communist Party came to
power. Finally, there has been a deep ambivalence
about western medicine. On the one hand, its benefits have been obvious, yet, on the other hand, the
vehicle by which it came to China is associated
with humiliation and weakness. This ambivalence
has been evident in the post-liberation era; doctors
periodically have been attacked as agents of western
"cultural imperialism."

THE LEGACY OF BASE AREA MEDICINE, 1927-1949

Perhaps the most important legacy of the past
was the medical system which the Chinese Communist
Party built during its long years of deprivation
and isolation in the South Kiangsi Soviet and
Yenan. The medical system which the Red Army built
in the 1930s and 1940s placed emphasis on prevention, on the use of paramedics with little formal
training, and on mass mobilization. These orientations became conspicuous facets of post-liberation
medical policy. These orientations assumed such
importance after 1949 partly because they resonated
well with the traditional importance attached to
prevention and partly because Red Army medicine had
had to adapt to manpower and resource scarcities
similar to those facing the regime after liberation.
The most important characteristic of the Red
Army's base area medical system was that it was
designed to treat wounded and prevent contagious
diseases from sapping the strength of soldiers.
The first communist hospital, Hsiao Ching I-yüan
(Little Well Hospital), was set up in late 1927, at
the newly established base at Chingkangshan. It
handled the wounded from the abortive Nanch'ang
Uprising and other encounters. While "hospital"
(i-yüan) may suggest a facility of some permanence
and sophistication, in fact, resources were virtually nonexistent. For instance, only traditional
Chinese pharmaceuticals were available to treat the
approximately 200 wounded who found their way
there.[29]
By the spring of 1931, the Chinese Communist
Party, which had become ensconced in the mountains
of southern Kiangsi Province, was facing the concerted attacks of the Kuomintang Army under Chiang
K'ai-shek. With casualties mounting, Dr. Ho Ch'eng,
later to become a major health policy-maker in the
1950s, was appointed to organize the General

11

Medical Department for the Worker-Peasant Red Army.
By 1934, under Ho's leadership, the General Medical
Department had expanded to the point where it ran
ten "rear area hospitals" (hou-fang i-yüan), each
of which allegedly had two "doctors" and a dozen or
so support personnel.[30]

The year after the founding of the General
Medical Department, Dr. Ho found it necessary to
establish a public health school; by the following
year, it was graduating approximately forty students
per annum. The students who were admitted generally
had primary school educations.[31] In the public
health school they were said to have been taught
the rudiments of internal medicine, surgery, pharmacology, and other subjects.

Despite these first halting efforts, base area
health conditions were appalling, a situation exacerbated by the increasingly effective Kuomintang
fourth and fifth "extermination" campaigns of 1932-
1934. In January 1934, the General Health Department issued a directive in which it instructed the
populace not to throw the bodies of the dead in
rivers and to purify all drinking water. During
this period, at least "several thousand" died of
dysentery each year.[32]

With the collapse of the South Kiangsi Soviet
in late 1934, all activities were ultimately moved
to the North, with the new focus of activity being
Yenan. While the cleanliness of Yenan presented a
sharp contrast to other places in China, medical
resources were tightly constrained. Once the anti-
Japanese War began in mid-1937, and the communist
base areas began to proliferate, the communists
faced the same problems they had encountered in the
South Kiangsi Soviet: an avalanche of casualties
and enormous threats to public health. Dr. Norman
Bethune, who had arrived in Yenan in early 1938,
described the medical conditions he found.

> We are now working in Hu Chia Ch'uan, a little
> village of about fifty houses. . . . There
> are 175 wounded here, scattered among the
> houses. This is what is meant by a "hospital"
> here. It would break your heart to see them
> lying on the brick k'angs with only a little
> straw beneath them. . . . The wounded are
> crawling with lice. . . . Three men, one with
> the loss of both feet through frost-bite
> gangrene, have no clothes at all to wear.[33]

While there is little specific information
presently available on the health situation in the
anti-Japanese base areas during the 1940s, it is
significant that 6 percent of the Shensi-Kansu-
Ninghsia Border Region's 1943 budget was allocated
to health care.[34] While this percentage is not
easily compared with post-liberation budgetary
figures (because of the military component to these
allocations), the communists never allocated more
than 2.6 percent of total budgetary expenditures to
health in the 1950-1956 period. As Selden observes,
even these relatively substantial efforts left many
sections of the base areas untouched,[35] not to mention the bulk of the country which was entirely
beyond communist control. As the communist-held
areas expanded rapidly in the mid and late 1940s,
the demands for medical care simply outstripped the
capacity of the army and the Chinese Communist Party
to meet them.

Only in the closing year of the revolution, as
major cities began to fall, did the communists begin
to acquire the basic infrastructure for a "mass"
curative health system, and even these facilities
had met the needs of only a minute fraction of the
urban population. As the units of the People's
Liberation Army rolled into the major cities in 1949,
an important encounter was shaping up, one that
provided a context for subsequent health politics.
The encounter centered around the question of what
kind of synthesis should occur between an urban-
oriented curative health system led by relatively
educated and professionalized medical doctors and
a guerrilla medical tradition which emphasized reliance upon mass mobilization, paramedics, and the
utilization of Chung-i. For the next twenty-eight
years, Chairman Mao Tse-tung became the biggest
promoter of the base area legacy.

THE HEALTH SITUATION AT LIBERATION AND CONDITIONS
TODAY

As Chairman Mao Tse-tung proclaimed the
founding of the People's Republic of China from
atop the Gate of Heavenly Peace in Peking on
October 1, 1949, he addressed a truly unhealthy
society. In China, as in other Third World countries, there was a detrimental synergism arising
from pervasive infection, malnutrition, inadequate
education, and poor environmental hygiene. The
cumulative effect of these problems fell with

13

particular force upon Chinese babies. The infant
mortality rate was approximately 200/1,000 live
births, a rate considerably higher than even India's
at the same time. Equally important, in the rice
growing areas of central and south China, the
vitality of the populace was drained by high rates
of parasitic diseases such as schistosomiasis
(with an estimated 10.5 million victims) and malaria
(with some areas having infection rates of 50 percent). Hookworm and kala-azar were enormous
problems as well, although there is an absence of
reliable statistical information. Contagious
diseases such as plague, cholera, and smallpox
were common, though we have no quantitative data
to indicate their frequency. Venereal disease was
exceptionally common, with prevalence rates of 3 to
5 percent in the cities and rates running as high
as 10 percent among the frontier peoples.[36]
      These high disease rates were, in part, a
reflection of the almost total absence of modern
medical resources and trained manpower. While one
ought not equate a system's capacity to promote
health with the availability of doctors and hospitals, statistical measures of these resources provide one vantage point from which to view the 1949
health situation. At liberation, China had between
10,000 and 20,000 trained medical doctors. This
means that there was one doctor for every 25,000-
50,000 persons. This ratio of doctors-to-popula-
tion is exceedingly low by any other standard than
abysmal poverty.[37] Hospital facilities were equally
scarce, with the province of Anhwei having .006
hospital beds per thousand population, Fukien
having .05, and the populous province of Shantung
having .06.[38] These are exceptionally low levels
of hospital facilities.
      Not only were hospital facilities most con-
spicuous by their rarity, those few resources which
did exist were concentrated in urban areas. For
instance, in 1949 Shanghai had 2.26 hospital beds
per thousand population and Canton had 2.11.[39]
Given the difficulties of travel and communication,
and given the absence of avenues of referral,
peasants generally were born and died without ever
having received modern medical attention.
      What is the situation in the mid-1970s, as
nearly as we can tell? While statistical data are
of uncertain reliability, even when available, both
the Chinese and visiting foreign medical personnel
agree that the situation has improved enormously.
In many ways, the People's Republic of China

14

provides an example of what can be done through fundamental organizational and social change. In 1959, the Chinese Medical Association announced that the national infant mortality rate had declined to 70/1,000 live births;[40] by the 1970s it is probably safe to say that it is below 60/1,000, though we only have scattered data.[41]

The post-liberation situation with respect to contagious diseases improved rapidly; smallpox, plague, and cholera were virtually eliminated by 1960.[42] Also, unlike India and Indonesia, once "eliminated," these diseases have apparently not reappeared, despite outbreaks in neighboring countries. Dealing with parasitic and water-borne diseases has proven much more difficult, because these maladies are built into the very fabric of a rice culture. The need to flood extensive areas, the continual human contact with infected water, and the use of human and animal excrement for fertilizer make it exceedingly difficult to eliminate hookworm, schistosomiasis, malaria, and other parasitic and water-borne diseases. Despite the difficulties, definite progress has been made in the reduction of schistosomiasis[43] and malaria. On a recent trip to the People's Republic, I was told that there were approximately 5,000 new cases of malaria in Shanghai during 1975; all of these new cases were concentrated in the ten rural counties. Typhoid is still a problem. While the frequency of the disease is generally unknown, Shanghai had about 600 cases in 1975. The most conspicuous indicator of Shanghai's progress was the fact that municipal health authorities now assert that the average life expectancy for females is 73.8 years and that for males is 69.3 years.[44] While these data must be viewed with caution, they indicate what is plain to see; the progress has been enormous, especially in coastal cities. Much still remains to be done, as well.

As noted above, in 1949 there were cavernous urban-rural and inter-provincial differentials in the distribution of curative health care. This problem was difficult to overcome when the emphasis of economic development throughout most of the 1950s was placed upon urban areas and the construction of a rather conventional city-based hospital system. It was structurally, economically, and politically difficult to imagine building curative facilities outside of an urban setting. Only in the post-Cultural Revolution period, when the emphasis has been placed upon developing a paramedic based medical care system, has there been identifiable movement toward equalization of access to medical care. Despite this, differentials in quality and access still favor relatively urbanized areas within provinces and relatively urbanized provinces. Several dramatic indications of this are available. For instance, in Peking and Shanghai I was told that all urban women give birth to their children in hospitals while all women in the surrounding counties give birth at home. Equally indicative of a persisting urban-rural gap is the fact that Shanghai municipal health authorities claim that the city's infant mortality rate is now 11.85/1,000 live births; the rate for surrounding Kiangsu Province is said to be 33.9/1,000 live births.[45]

THE PRE-1949 LEGACY AS ONE CONTEXT FOR POST-1949 POLICY-MAKING

Throughout the remainder of this study the reader should be struck by the degree to which the pre-1949 legacy has shaped post-liberation medical policy. Mao Tse-tung's emphasis on preventive medical care was the stock and trade of traditional medical practitioners for thousands of years before him. The post-1949 ambivalence toward western-style medicine, and the concentration of medical resources in urban areas, were two important residues of missionary medicine in the nineteenth and twentieth centuries. The continual conflict between traditional and modern medicine in the post-1949 period has roots into the previous century. Finally, the emphasis upon paramedic medicine and the mobilization of laymen in mass health campaigns was the hallmark of the Red Army's medical system in the 1930s and 1940s. In brief, the story of post-1949 medical policy-making is importantly the story of how these acquired predispositions and patterns of behavior affected the way in which problems were perceived and potential solutions identified.

NOTES

1. Ilza Veith, The Yellow Emperor's Classic of Internal Medicine (Berkeley: University of California Press, 1970), pp. 4-9.

2. Veith, pp. 58-76; Felix Mann, Acupuncture (New York: Vintage Books, 1972).

3.   Lee T'ao, "A Brief History of Obstetrics and Gynecology in China from Ancient Times to Before the Opium War," Chinese Medical Journal 77 (1958):478.

4.   Ralph C. Croizier, Traditional Medicine in Modern China (Cambridge: Harvard University Press, 1968), pp. 19-20.

5.   Lee T'ao, "Chinese Medicine During the Ming Dynasty (1368-1644 A.D.)," Chinese Medical Journal 76 (1958):180-181.

6.   John Z. Bowers, "Surgery Past and Present," in Medicine and Public Health in the People's Republic of China, ed., Joseph R. Quinn (Washington, D.C.: National Institutes of Health, 1972), pp. 55-56; Croizier, p. 25.

7.   Lee T'ao, "Chinese Medicine During the Chin (1127-1234) and Yüan (1234-1368) Eras," Chinese Medical Journal 73 (1955):242.

8.   Croizier, p. 26.

9.   Croizier, pp. 27-28.

10.   Lee T'ao, "Chinese Medicine During the Chin," p. 255.

11.   Hsin Jen Wei [New people's health] (Peking: People's Health Press, 1967).

12.   Jonathan Spence, To Change China (Boston: Little, Brown & Company, 1969), pp. 34-56.

13.   W. H. Medhurst, China: Its State and Prospects (Boston: London Missionary Society, 1838).

14.   Mao Tse-tung, "In Memory of Norman Bethune," in Selected Works of Mao Tse-tung, vol. 2 (Peking: Foreign Languages Press, 1965), pp. 337-338.

15.   Mao Tse-tung, "The Chinese Revolution and the Chinese Communist Party," in Selected Works of Mao Tse-tung, vol. 2 (Peking: Foreign Languages Press, 1965), p. 312.

16.   Mary E. Ferguson, China Medical Board and Peking Union Medical College (New York: China Medical Board, 1970), p. 22; John Z. Bowers, Western Medicine in a Chinese Palace (New York: Josiah Macy, Jr. Foundation, 1972).

17. Pierre Huard and Ming Wong, Chinese Medicine
(Toronto: McGraw-Hill Book Company, 1968), pp.
158-159.

18. Wu Lien-teh, Plague Fighter: Autobiography of
a Chinese Physician (Cambridge: W. Heffer & Sons,
1959).

19. Croizier, p. 87.

20. Robert Worth, "Institution Building in the
People's Republic of China: The Rural Health
Centre," unpublished manuscript, p. 6.

21. Lu Hsun, "Medicine," in Selected Stories of Lu
Hsun (Peking: Foreign Languages Press, 1972), pp.
25-33.

22. Croizier, pp. 129-130.

23. Mao Tse-tung, "The United Front in Cultural
Work," in Selected Works of Mao Tse-tung, vol. 3
(Peking: Foreign Languages Press, 1965), p. 236.

24. Huard and Wong, p. 159

25. Ferguson, p. 58.

26. C. C. Chen, "Public Health in Rural Reconstruc-
tion at Ting Hsien," Annual Report (Department of
Public Health, Chinese National Association of the
Mass Education Movement, 1934); Sidney D. Gamble,
Ting Hsien (Stanford: Stanford University Press,
1968).

27. William Y. Chen, "Medicine and Public Health,"
China Quarterly, no. 6 (1961), p. 154.

28. Croizier, p. 249.

29. Tai Cheng-hua, "Chung-kuo Jen-min Chieh-fang-
chün Tsai Ti Erh T'se Kuo-nei Ko-ming Chan-cheng
Shih-ch'i Te Wei-sheng Kung-tso Tsu-chih Ch'ing-
k'uang" [The situation of health organization of
the Chinese People's Liberation Army during the
period of the Second Revolutionary Civil War],
I-hsüeh Shih Yü Pao-chien Tsu-chih [The history of
medicine and health organization], no. 1 (1958), p.
34.

30. Tai Cheng-hua, p. 35.

31. Tai Cheng-hua, p. 36.

32. Tai Cheng-hua, p. 37.

33. Ted Allen and Sydney Gordon, The Scalpel, the Sword: The Story of Doctor Norman Bethune (Toronto: McClelland and Stewart, Ltd., 1972), p. 193.

34. Jerome Ch'ên, Mao and the Chinese Revolution (London: Oxford University Press, 1965), p. 206.

35. Mark Selden, The Yenan Way (Cambridge: Harvard University Press, 1972), p. 268.

36. David M. Lampton, Health, Conflict, and the Chinese Political System, Michigan Papers in Chinese Studies, no. 18 (Ann Arbor: Center for Chinese Studies, 1974), pp. 2-4.

37. John Bryant, Health and the Developing World (Ithaca: Cornell University Press, 1969), p. 51

38. David M. Lampton, "Performance and the Chinese Political System: A Preliminary Assessment of Education and Health Policies" (Paper delivered at the 1975 Annual Meeting of the American Political Science Association, San Francisco, California, September 2-5, 1975), p. 41.

39. David M. Lampton, "Performance," p. 41.

40. Chu Fu-t'ang, "Accomplishments in Child Health Since Liberation," Chinese Medical Journal 79 (1959):385.

41. Lampton, "Performance," p. 62.

42. Lampton, "Performance," p. 62.

43. "Report of the American Schistosomiasis Delegation to the People's Republic of China," obtainable from the National Academy of Sciences, Committee on Scholarly Communications with the People's Republic of China, Washington, D.C.

44. David M. Lampton, "Administration of the Pharmaceutical, Research, Public Health, and Population Bureaucracies," forthcoming from the National Academy of Sciences, Committee on Scholarly Communications with the People's Republic of China, Washington, D.C. (1977).

45. "Child Health Care in New China," <u>Chinese Medical Journal</u> 1 (1975): 91.

Chapter 2
CONSOLIDATION OF POWER AND PROFESSIONAL DOMINANCE: THE DOCTORS IN CHARGE (1949-1954)

INTRODUCTION

Initial health policy reflected the importance of three factors: One was the dominance of independently-minded professionals from the People's Liberation Army and elite medical schools in the policy-making system. Secondly, the Ministry of Public Health's (Wei-sheng-pu) definition of the situation affected outcomes. Finally, financial allocations to the Ministry of Public Health were small because the revenue producing capabilities of the regime were limited and because the military required huge appropriations in order to finish the civil war, restore order, and fight the Korean War. The way in which these factors interacted to produce medical policies is the story to which we now turn.

POLICY-MAKING LEADERSHIP: STABILITY AND CHANGE

As the dust settled in the immediate post-takeover period, governmental and Party functions at the local level were vested in Military Affairs Control Commissions (Chün-shih Kuan-chih Wei-yüan-hui).[1] Nationally, by September 1949, the "Organic Law of the People's Republic of China" established the framework for a formally coalition government. While there were substantial variations in the rapidity with which Military Affairs Control Commissions relinquished authority to newly staffed government organs, by the convening of the August 1950 First National Health Conference, most areas had functioning health bureaus and the Wei-sheng-pu had been operational for nearly a year.
While both the Party and the Government lacked expert cadres, the government apparatus could more

easily rectify this problem than the Party. It was
more difficult to build a politically reliable vanguard organization than to construct a moderately
dependable administrative structure. These differences showed up in the recruitment of Ministry of
Public Health personnel.

Once the Wei-sheng-pu's structure had congealed,
at least six vice-ministerial posts had to be filled,
bureau heads had to be found, directors for semi-
independent units under the Ministry had to be
appointed, and leadership for five units outside,
but subordinate to, the Ministry had to be located.[2]
In addition, the six administrative regions (into
which China was divided until 1954), the provinces,
and all of the counties had similar bureaucracies.
Finally, the Chinese Academy of Sciences (Chung-kuo
K'o-hsüeh-yüan) needed leadership, and the myriad
of hospitals and medical schools had to be staffed.
With only a pool of from ten to twenty thousand
western-style physicians to draw upon, the government could not make political criteria paramount.

Doctors who had served in the army were
recruited into the highest Wei-sheng-pu positions.
These doctors, in their wartime capacities in an
over-burdened medical system, had been relatively
free from Party control. Questions of political
vs. professional control had rarely arisen because
of the manifest constraints of the wartime situation. The doctors who assumed leading roles in
1949, then, had been nurtured in an environment in
which their professional values had never really
come into conflict with the revolutionary dictates
of the Party's political apparatus. This was to
change! Who were these individuals, how did they
relate to the medical profession, and what relationship do these facts have to subsequent policies?

In 1950, Dr. Fu Lien-chang was appointed
president of the Chinese Medical Association (hereafter CMA), an appendage of the Ministry of Public
Health. Fu was a respected doctor and this fact,
alone, reduced some fears. During the revolution,
Fu had been in charge of Fu Yin (Good Tidings)
Hospital in Fukien Province, had been a leading
figure in the Red Army hospital system,[3] and was
credited with saving Mao's life.[4] Further consoli-
dating Fu's position as an intermediary between the
government and the medical profession was his appointment as vice-minister of public health in
April 1952.

Fu was not the only initial appointee to the
health bureaucracy who was congenial to the

22

western-style medical profession. In December 1949,
Dr. Ho Ch'eng was appointed first vice-minister of
public health. During the revolution, Ho had been
the director of the General Medical Department of
the Red Army. As first vice-minister, Ho had
responsibility for the day-to-day operation of the
Ministry of Public Health. In addition, Su Ching-
kuan was given a vice-ministerial portfolio in 1949.
Su had been the first western-style physician to
join the Red Army and had been involved with public
health education.[5]

Those persons named to lead health work in each
of the six administrative regions were western-
style physicians as well. When the regions were
abolished (1954), many of these individuals were
elevated to vice-ministerial posts in the Wei-sheng-
pu. Dr. Ch'ien Hsin-chung was in charge of health
work in the Southwest Military Affairs Commission
(1950); he had been director of the 15th Army Corps'
Public Health Bureau.[6] In the East China Region,
Dr. Tsui I-t'ien was director of the Public Health
Department and simultaneously director of the
Shanghai Municipal Health Bureau. Tsui had been
trained in western medicine in Shengyang; he moved
to Peking in 1954 and was elevated to a vice-ministerial post.[7] Similarly, Dr. Ho Piao (Ho Lung's
adopted son) was initially appointed head of health
work in the Northwest Military Affairs Region. Like
Tsui, he became a vice-minister of public health in
1954.[8]

The final Ministry appointment of immediate
interest was Li Teh-ch'uan; she became minister of
public health. The reason for mentioning Li last
is that she was the least important major personality. Li, the wife of Feng Yu-hsiang, was brought
into the Wei-sheng-pu as a united front personage.
She rarely exerted, or sought to exert, much
authority.

Below the vice-ministerial level, ten major
bureaus were staffed. Some, like the Bureau of
Drugs (Yao-cheng-chü) and the Bureau of Contagious
Diseases (Wei-sheng Fang-i-chü), were predominantly
manned by medical experts; others (e.g., the Personnel Bureau) were staffed exclusively by Party
nonprofessionals. In general, the more technical
the responsibility of the bureau the more dominant
were professionals. The power of bureau heads was
at its apex during this period because each had the
authority to independently contact and direct health
units at the regional, provincial, and county
levels.[9]

The Party leadership dimension. The analyst of communist systems would normally expect that the foregoing list of leaders omits the most important actors of all; Party political cadres. Because the Party apparatus lacked the trained and reliable manpower to make its control either effective or pervasive, the organizational role of the Party was down-played in this period. Schurmann suggests, "Vertical rule reached a high point around 1954. Not only the major economic, but other ministries as well, had created nation-wide networks of organization."[10]

Because the Party lacked effective administrative control over the Ministry, Mao periodically "attacked" the Wei-sheng-pu, hoping to bring his values to bear on the policies being churned out. The Chairman employed this tactic twice in 1953 and once again in 1954. On April 3, 1953, Mao blasted the Ministry saying,

> The disclosure by Comrade Pai xx made me think of whether there is any major difference between the leadership work of the government health departments and that of the army's health departments. I suspect that the leadership work of the government health departments is in the same mess as that of the army's health departments.[11]

At an October 1953 Politburo meeting, Mao lashed out at the Wei-sheng-pu's leadership for deferring to professional opinion.[12] Finally (winter 1954), the Chairman spoke at the Central Committee and condemned the Ministry's failure to follow the mandate of the First National Health Conference with respect to traditional Chinese medicine (Chung-i).[13]

LEADERSHIP'S EVALUATION OF THE PROBLEMS

Not only the identity and background of leaders shaped policy, but so did their evaluations of the problems. How did these individuals weigh health care relative to other social needs and how did they order priorities within the health sphere?

The most interesting question (How are funds allocated between public health and other areas of social responsibility?) is an obscure dimension of the policy process. Available information suggests that this was (and is) an ad hoc process in which major ministry officials, State Council members,

and Party figures sit down and set relative priorities. This, in turn, suggests that informal patterns of influence were decisive in determining outcomes. Who was invited to these discussions, their
viewpoints, and their relative weight, are unknown.
We do know, however, that in 1949 and 1950 the
amount of money allocated to health care suggests
that, in comparison to the needs of the military and
the economy, it received relatively low priority.
Health care received 1.0 percent of total government
expenditure in comparison to defense which received
41.5 percent.[14]
        Within the health sphere, the objective prob-
lems were enormous. Kuo Mo-jo noted that the
immediate rural health task of 1949-1952 was the
halting of epidemic diseases.[15] This could be
accomplished with a relatively low investment in
fixed-site clinics. In the minority areas, the
difficulties were staggering and made all the more
pressing by the regime's desire to exert control
over terrain that had been only nominally under
Chinese domination for over a hundred years. Hu
Ch'uan-k'uei, a famous dermatologist and later
president of Peking Medical College, was sent to
the northwest to survey conditions there.

        The rates both of incidence of disease and of
        mortality in the region are extremely high.
        The incidence of venereal diseases, both
        syphilis and gonorrhea, runs from 40-70 per-
        cent or even higher in many areas. Smallpox,
        diphtheria, typhus fever, and measles are
        common, as are thyroid trouble, leprosy, kala-
        azar, pneumonia, and vitamin deficiencies.
        Resistance to tuberculosis is notably low in
        Sinkiang. Infant mortality rates are often
        over 65 percent.[16]

        Urban medical problems were substantially dif-
ferent. Epidemic diseases were less evident and
chronic debilitating difficulties more apparent.
Tuberculosis was a serious problem which required
extensive capital investment to treat. Also, previous institution building had been concentrated in
the cities. What little capital was available
seemed most appropriately spent in restoring pre-
existent facilities to full capacity.
        The Ministry of Public Health faced another
problem in the cities. Demand for curative health
care was growing rapidly. This was partly due to
the sudden coverage of 3.3 million workers under the

Insurance Act of 1951.[17] By 1953, the number of
insured had reached 4.8 million, in addition to an
unknown number of Party and government cadres who
became entitled to free medical care (kung-fei i-
liao). With the removal of financial barriers for
a substantial number of urbanites, clinics became
overcrowded.[18] Compounding the problem, because
urban incomes were growing more rapidly than those
in rural areas, even urbanites who were not entitled
to free or insured treatment could more easily
imagine paying for services than their country
cousins. In short, the effective demand for curative care was concentrated in the cities.

    Because patient loads were large, the Ministry
was continually besieged with requests from county
hospitals for more money. When the Wei-sheng-pu
said "no," local administrators were prone to say,
as in fact one in Lien P'ing Hsien did, "Other
people just do not understand the budgetary difficulties of the hospital."[19] Other complaints
deluging the Ministry concerned patient dissatisfaction with the quality and speed of service, fraudu-
lent drug charges, and high prices.[20] The Ministry
faced contradictory demands for better, quicker,
and cheaper service from patients and requests for
subsidies from local health institutions. At the
same time, it was constrained by its incapacity to
adequately increase its share of the national budget.

MINISTRY RESOURCES AND ANTICIPATED RESISTANCES

    Financial constraints are the bane of most
bureaucrats and this was certainly the case for the
Wei-sheng-pu leadership. The Ministry's 1950 budget
was 71 million yüan (hereafter ¥); this rose to 163
million ¥ in 1951, 374 million ¥ in 1952, and 565
million ¥ in 1953.[21] Even in 1953, this represented
only .96¥ per capita (or about 44¢ U.S.). Added
responsibilities offset even this meager increase
in resources.[22] The introduction of free and
insured coverage for millions of Chinese workers
and cadres increased Ministry burdens, even though
union funds did defray an unknown percentage of the
added increment of expense. Consequently, the
Ministry had to rely upon non-budgetary sources of
capital if the scope of its activities was to be
expanded.

    Private physician capital represented one
resource. Physicians had their own offices,
pharmacies, and practices; rationalizing these

dispersed facilities was one way to expand services. In July 1951, the Ministry inaugurated the policy of establishing united clinics (lien-ho chen-so), or group practices. Doctors were encouraged to consolidate their practices, build shared facilities, and regulate fees.

> The initial funds were collected from the doctors who subscribed shares of capital as their financial conditions permitted. Medical equipment was also pooled by the doctors, part of which was accepted in lieu of cash capital and part was on loan on a temporary basis. It was also agreed upon that 40 percent of the monthly income will be set apart for business expansion, 30 percent will be salaries for working personnel, and 30 percent will be reserved as dividends for shareholders.[23]

Another asset which the Ministry had was the initial symmetry of its goals and those of the western-style medical community. For years, the Chinese Medical Association (CMA) had encouraged the establishment of a strong and centralized health administration that would be capable of genuinely improving public health. Of course, China's western-style doctors did not look upon the communist assumption of power with complete lack of concern, but, they were generally willing to cooperate, as their June 1949 policy program indicates. Five objectives were established in the CMA's "Outline of Plans of Future Medical Work in China": (1) ". . . all the medical and pharmaceutical enterprises will gradually diverge from private and commercial ownership leading to the final goal of State Medicine." (2) "The object of medical training is for: Scientific thinking, Spirit of service, and Technical progress, all three are of equal importance." (3) "For the practicability of medical training, two grade systems of Medical Center are to be adopted . . . stressing equally upon the teaching and research as well as service . . ." (4) "The unscientific native medicine is to be reoriented and duly abolished." (5) "The patent medicine and drugs for advertisement should be strictly controlled and abolished."[24] In sum, the CMA was not opposed to "state medicine" as long as quality was maintained and research continued. Only the medical profession's attitude toward traditional medicine was to produce major friction from the start.

27

As the Wei-sheng-pu leaders surveyed the horizon for solutions to their problems, the Soviet Union loomed large. The Russian medical system had an integrated spectrum of health personnel ranging from health workers in rural areas to highly trained specialists in polyclinics. This was certainly consistent with the base area legacy already discussed. As Fu Lien-chang summed up a few years later, "In short, the organizational systems, methods of work, scientific theories and technology in Soviet medicine are what we learn from the Soviet Union."[25] In addition, Moscow was willing to send medical specialists to China. As Minister Li Teh-ch'uan and Vice-Minister Ho Ch'eng told the State Council in 1950, "Our leading health organizations promoted and organized temporary medical teams with the help of Soviet health specialists."[26]

One of the Wei-sheng-pu's greatest assets was the presence of an urban medical infrastructure. According to Chen, at the end of World War II China had over 1,700 county health centers, 26 provincial centers, 125 provincial clinics, 307 missionary facilities, 317 nursing schools, and 22 midwifery schools.[27] By the end of 1951, there were 1,865 county health centers.[28]

Reinforcing the logic of maximizing utilization of existent resources and the desire of health professionals to consolidate health institutions in urban areas, was the fact that health care was explicitly linked with increased industrial production. It was felt that healthy workers were more productive. Heavy industrial workers were the first (and only) laboring group to become entitled to comprehensive health coverage. The policy of concentrating curative facilities in urban areas was made explicit when New China News Agency announced (1953), "In the field of health work, medical and health institutions in cities and in factories and mines and along the railways will be expanded and new ones added."[29]

The view of the Ministry to emerge from the foregoing is that of an organization with substantial independence (of the Party political apparatus) and a leadership which possessed medical and military experience. While the leadership, formally, had almost unlimited policy discretion, in reality, the limits on choice were severe. The dearth of money, the need to maintain an already existent urban infrastructure, the influence of Soviet advisors, and professional pressures to which the leadership was responsive, all reduced latitude.

Also, the policies of other agencies were significant, but only marginally under the Ministry's control. Economic plans, budgetary allocations, the
price and volume of pharmaceuticals, and the expansion of the size of the insured population were all
areas of vital concern to the Ministry but were
decisions over which it had relatively little control. In short, the Ministry faced enormous problems and its options were few.

HEALTH POLICIES, 1949-1954

     Medical education policy was a reflection of
leadership aspirations moderated by objective
problems, social pressures, and a paucity of political and economic resources. The regime's educational plan was unveiled at the First National
Health Conference (August 1950) and was virtually
identical with the program which the CMA had proposed in mid-1949. The educational structure was
to have three tiers: five-year higher training,
greatly expanded middle-level medical education,
and accelerated production of "health workers."[30]
     Kuo Mo-jo and Dr. Ho Ch'eng, speaking to the
CMA in August 1951, both tried to reassure the
assembled doctors that no contradiction between
expanded medical education and their desires for
"quality" needed to exist.

     Through the intensification of scientific and
     research activities it has been possible both
     to raise the standard of medical education
     and make it more widespread.[31]

The effort to make medical knowledge more widespread
was not to be permitted to impede quality. For
example, China Union Medical College kept its
admission standards as rigorous as ever, requiring
a three-year pre-medical course before the appli-
cant could take the entrance examination.[32] In
addition, major (full-length) medical schools were
insulated from the burden of having to train lower-
level medical personnel; county hospitals were
given the responsibility for training such individuals.[33]
     Educational policy reflected the strong insti-
tutional position of western-style physicians and
the kinds of inputs solicited at the First National
Health Conference. That conference was dominated
by medical doctors. Educational guidelines were

29

almost a word-for-word copy of the CMA's pre-liberation proposals. Secondly, physicians were conspicuous in the Ministry's Medical Education Bureau
(I-hsüeh Chiao-yü-szu).[34] The only bureau for
traditional medicine was in the Ministry of Commerce
(Shang-yeh-pu), meaning that traditional practitioners had almost no institutional leverage over
health policy. Finally, the Wei-sheng-pu gave
important positions to Soviet medical professionals;
they were particularly evident in the Medical Education Bureau. Under their influence, there was a
strong tendency to replicate the Soviet model which
stressed expertise.

We conclude that leadership composition and the
organization of the Ministry (which excluded traditional practitioners and included Soviet specialists)
limited the range of inputs and skewed policy.
Financial pressures, as we shall see shortly, made
it imperative that the counties assume most of the
burden for training middle level personnel. Only
medical education in the major schools was the
direct responsibility of the Wei-sheng-pu.

Medical research guidelines reflected the same
political and social forces. In fact, the two were
intimately linked with the assertion that better
research led to better education.[35] In July 1952,
scientific research was given a boost by Ch'en Po-ta
who said, research should ". . . serve definite
purposes and lead to the solution of important problems of a mass character."[36] The CMA's Fu Lien-
chang outlined the research tasks as he saw them.
"We must raise the standard of medical research and
emphasize the importance of research in relationship
to practical needs."[37] Both Ch'en and Fu, in
slightly different ways to be sure, gave a large
and legitimate role to medical research.

The western-style medical profession encouraged
this trend. Dr. C. U. Lee, of China Union Medical
College, gave a glowing account of the college's
research program since liberation.

> Dr. Lee stated that the college is building up
> scientific research with the practical needs of
> the people. Since 1953, he continued, 203
> research items have been undertaken. . . . Next
> year the research program will include 267
> items. They include the study of higher ner-
> vous activity, effects of excitation and inhi-
> bition of the cerebral cortex, the study of
> living substance of noncellular form, tumors,
> cancer, internal secretion, and other clinical
> problems.[38]

The question which arises is, why did medical research trends maintain such continuity with pre-liberation policy? Besides the fact that the Party lacked sufficient manpower and expertise to make its control effective, Party policy was not significantly different from governmental actions. In addition, no comprehensive research program was formulated until 1956-1957; in the absence of concrete policy alternatives, events moved in the direction of their previous momentum.

The very structure of the Ministry also contributed to continuity in research. The Ministry's Scientific Committee of Medical Sciences (I-hsüeh K'o-hsüeh Wei-yüan-hui) was highly influential in determining research priorities during this period. One interviewee described the committee and its duties.

> It has a chief and five staff members who are all doctors of western medicine, mostly women. There are no Party members in this department except the chief. The important qualification for these staff members is their medical knowledge and skill. The department discusses the medical research to be carried out throughout China. It decides which hospitals shall do research and on what lines research is to be carried out. [39]

A detailed knowledge of these individuals, and the resources at their command, is unavailable. However, the expected biases of such professionals seem to be reflected in research policy during this period.* In addition, a substantial portion of all medical research was carried out under the auspices of the Chinese Academy of Sciences; much was not funded through the Ministry at all.

Health delivery policy reflected economic constraints and the different health problems facing medical authorities in various sections of the country. In rural areas, the county hospital was to be the focus of cure, prevention, and training, with "prevention first." In coastal areas in central and south China, the county health system was already rather well developed,[40] whereas in north China there was comparatively less infrastructure to build on. In the western areas, little work had been done at all. In order to cope with such disparities, the six administrative regions were given

---

*See Appendix B, for content analysis of research appearing in the Chinese Medical Journal.

substantial autonomy in designing policies to meet
the needs of their areas.

The relative independence of these regional
bureaus tended to accentuate the impact of western-
style doctors. Each regional health bureau had one
at its head. The close local proximity of these
regional health leaders made them vulnerable to local
professional influence. Apparently such influence
was effective because in March 1953, Tsui I-t'ien,
the director of the East China Region's Public Health
Department, was denounced for his reliance upon professional advice in the formulation of regional
health policy.[41] The result of regional decentralization appears to have been to make health delivery
policy more responsive to the local situation and
professional demands.

In general, counties were in charge of retraining
old-style midwives, health workers, and giving inoculations in the countryside.[42] The vehicles for ac-
complishing most of these tasks were roving health
teams, usually operating from the county seat.
These teams made substantial progress in immunizing
the population against contagious diseases, but
problems did exist.

> Summarizing the work of the past six months, one
> finds shortcomings. In the preventive work for
> contagious diseases, the report on occurrences
> has not been sufficiently careful and alert,
> while the city has discriminated against the
> suburbs.[43]

Urban delivery policy had to deal with a somewhat different set of problems. Because population
was concentrated, the task of inoculating urbanites
was completed in relatively short order. The next
task was curing those who were already ill and had
chronic problems. Old hospitals were expanded and
new ones built as rapidly as local finances would
permit. As an example, because Peking had a large
and relatively substantial tax base, this task was
accomplished more rapidly than could be the case in
less prosperous areas.[44] Canton, Peking, and Shanghai
witnessed a growth of hospital facilities that outstripped that going on anywhere else. The disease
picture, location of pre-existent facilities, distribution of wealth, and the emphasis on heavy industry
all produced an initial urban bias in the delivery
of health care. Of course, these initial "temporary"
measures created constituencies which, in the future,
would resist change.

Not only were cities in a better position to supply curative services, they also faced a larger effective demand. In 1952, 4 million persons were entitled to free medical care, most of whom were in cities.[45] The increase in urban demand was so enormous that publicly-run facilities were incapable of meeting the wave. "Private" clinics were pressed into service and given responsibility for meeting the needs of entire factories. In Tientsin, even in 1955, such clinics were handling 21 percent of the municipality's patient load.[46]

Concluding, curative institutions were primarily in the towns. In rural areas, the delegation of so many tasks to a unit of government with relatively little financial base (the county) meant that prevention would have had to be emphasized as the only alternative to no health care. Equally important, the most "valued" sector (in a developmental sense) of the population was in the cities. Finally, because of the physician shortage, it made a great deal of sense to concentrate scarce manpower where it could simultaneously treat patients, conduct research, and teach; this was synonymous with urban teaching hospitals.

Finances are an essential part of the explanation for the shape of health programs. Every directive was formulated in such a way as to reduce the economic liabilities of central and regional health organs. A crucial bureaucratic game was being played in which taxation was an important element.

Tzu-ch'ou [self help] refers to hsien level and below revenue which the center does not control; it is decided upon by the local authorities, in an independent search for revenue. . . . Each hsien was able to levy an uncontrolled amount to help meet the costs of programs it was expected to implement. . . . Tzu-ch'ou, then, could be looked upon as a sort of a squeeze. The sources of revenue were the same as the regular tax. Local units were given more tasks than revenue to meet these tasks, and were told that they must think of a method.[47]

With these taxation arrangements as a backdrop, the April 1950 health directive, placing substantial burdens on the county, assumes new meaning. Because the Ministry's budget was relatively small, as noted, it was inconceivable that it could pay for all that needed to be done. It was in the Wei-sheng-pu's interest to give county organs as many responsibilities as possible and to let them extract the

33

necessary resources. The county's interest, on the other hand, was to limit burdens, raise charges and ask for central subsidy.[48] As a consequence of these pressures, reports periodically appeared alleging that county facilities often overcharged for drugs[49] and charged excessive fees. The open-ended taxation system tended to alienate the rural populace as well.[50]

In large urban areas, the financial situation was different, though each administrative level was supposed to be maximally self-sufficient. Because of the already substantial "private" health infrastructure, local authorities could control hospital fees without having to assume immediate responsibility for the operation of all facilities. In effect, the authorities could substitute private for public capital; this alternative was unavailable in rural areas and small county towns. Secondly, because most western-style doctors were in the cities, united clinics tended to be similarly concentrated.

For all these reasons, then, private fee-for-service practice continued, with relatively little obstruction, until 1954.

> In the years up to 1954, private doctors could charge extremely high fees for their services and an operation could cost anything from a few hundred to over 2,000 dollars. By 1956, however, the doctors were questioned closely on fees they charged for their services. . . .[51]

Sizable trade union health and welfare funds augmented the aggregate amount of urban health resources. While no reliable statistics bearing on the size of these monies exist, their magnitude was probably substantial. In many cases, industrial enterprises built their own hospitals, clinics, and sanatoria, almost wholly beyond the Ministry of Public Health's control.[52] In those cases when union monies were spent in the regular hospital system, it appears that local administrators occasionally had the incentive to overcharge insured workers in order to make up operating losses in dealing with other categories of patients.[53] One strategy which was open to health administrators, then, was for them to transfer financial burdens to the industrial enterprises.

Summing up, urban areas not only had a much greater revenue base, they also had a greater capacity to substitute private for public capital. The Ministry's major objective was to meet the needs

of the most people with the least expenditure of
its resources. Given this objective, financial
responsibility had to be given to the localities.
This meant, in turn, that prosperous areas could
expand their curative systems much more rapidly
than less fortunate localities. In addition, decentralization of revenue generating and collecting
authority gave rise to local abuses which, eventu-
ally, would be dealt with in the tax reform of 1958.
In short, the financial imperatives of the early
1950s necessitated actions which created, or maintained, a rural-urban gap and which gave rise to
substantial abuses.[54] At the time, however, there
appeared to be no other alternative.

Policy regarding the conditions of physician
employment. The position of physicians maintained
continuity with the past. The staffs of major
medical facilities, from the presidents to the
department heads, remained largely the same. Doctors continued to be preeminent in the medical
hierarchy. Preventive work in the mobile medical
teams was under their leadership. Only in 1951 and
1952 did doctors experience significant criticism
during the "thought reform" (szu-hsiang kai-tsao)
campaign. Generally, this movement was a "gentle
rain"; it focused almost exclusively upon famous
physicians who had had close relationships with the
"imperialists" (e.g., C. U. Lee of China Union
Medical College). The Korean War without doubt
exacerbated these latent tensions. This campaign,
however, never turned into a general assault upon
physicians; even those individuals attacked by name
remained at their jobs.

The significant question is, why were physicians so apparently successful in insulating themselves? One reason was that many physicians were
in policy-making positions themselves. In the
absence of outside (the profession) control, it
would be unlikely that doctors would divest their
fellow professionals of influence. Secondly, doctors had resources which the regime needed and
which would be most efficiently utilized if compliance were voluntary. Thirdly, the Soviet Union's
experience accentuated the role of doctors and
almost all of the Soviet advisors to the Ministry
were physicians. Finally, the objectives of the
health leadership were not significantly different
from those of the medical community at large.

Strangely enough, policy vis à vis traditional
practitioners proved to be the vortex of political
controversy. The reception accorded traditional

35

doctors was quite different from that given the western school. Even though Mao had called for the "union" of traditional and western medicine in 1944,[55] 1950,[56] and 1953,[57] the position of the Ministry, the CMA, and some high-ranking Party members, such as Kuo Mo-jo, was one of implicit (if not explicit) opposition, as mentioned in Chapter 1.

The "correct" policy with respect to Chung-i was to be "union and reform." Behind this slogan, however, there were disagreements over how much "reform" and how much "union" were appropriate. The Ministry emphasized "reform" while Mao under-lined "union." In March 1950, Minister of Public Health Li Teh-ch'uan told a group of leading traditional doctors that they would have to improve their techniques and to this end the China Medical Improvement Academy would be established. The Ministry's May 1951 directive stated, "Because of this [Chung-i's lack of scientific foundation] Chung-i must endeavor to incorporate the knowledge of scientific medicine and improve its methods of treatment."[58]

Simultaneously, a second area of controversy arose. In what sense were "united clinics" to be united? Should these clinics merely be group practices or should they also be the vehicles for bringing about the union of Chinese and western medicine? Because western-style physicians were usually employed in urban hospitals, it was rural traditional practitioners who were predominantly encouraged to form united clinics. Those western-style practitioners who did build group practices generally formed groups with no traditional part-ners.[59] In short, united clinics did not overcome the divisions between the two medical traditions.

Traditional medical research was no less a subject of controversy. The First National Health Conference had proposed that Chung-i research centers be built; in fact, none were constructed until 1955.[60] One reason was that the Chinese Academy of Sciences was responsible for establishing broad research priorities; no traditional practitioner held a major position in the Academy. Also, the Ministry's Scientific Committee on Medical Science was completely dominated by western-style doctors, as noted earlier. In short, within the science policy-making apparatus, traditional physicians were exceptionally weak. In China, as elsewhere, the capacity to achieve parochial interests is dependent upon institutional leverage.

The foregoing suggests that Chung-i's position was in jeopardy in the early 1950s. Just how precarious that status was became clear in April 1953, when the Wei-sheng-pu set up a National Examination Committee for Health Workers. At the head of the committee was Wang Pin, the head of public health in north China. Wang had recently written articles labelling traditional medicine "feudal." NCNA outlined the committee's mission in forthright terms.

> The present number of medical and health personnel falls far short of needs while among the people there are large numbers of medical and health personnel graduated from unofficial medical schools and lacking proper qualifications.[61]

The origins of policy toward Chung-i are complex. One reason for its vulnerability was its institutional weakness within the policy-making apparatus; it had no bureau in the Ministry of Public Health and it played little, if any, role in the Chinese Academy of Sciences. Secondly, western-style doctors were overwhelmingly dominant in the health system at the national, regional, and local levels. In 1949, the CMA had called for the abolition of traditional medicine. Thirdly, given the Ministry's priorities of encouraging research, giving inoculations, and restoring and expanding curative and educational institutions, western-style doctors seemed more relevant. In addition, even dedicated revolutionaries like Kuo Mo-jo were ambivalent about the scientific value, and ideological costs, of Chung-i. Finally, given the financial constraints of the early 1950s, it made little sense to many to invest scarce resources in something with such an apparently small payoff.

SUMMARY

Initially, the Wei-sheng-pu was quite independent of the Party political apparatus, being staffed with western-style doctors who had army experience. Their professional and military backgrounds made them resistant to the imposition of political controls. Limited Party capability to make "dual rule" effective meant that the bulk of the explanation for health policy lay in the Ministry and its subsidiary organs.

Because the Ministry of Public Health was the primary source of health policy, its leadership, its institutional structure, the leadership's perceptions, and the available resources, determined policy. In soliciting advice and formulating policy, the doctors in charge of the Ministry primarily relied upon the opinions of other professionals. The result? The policy guidelines of the First National Health Conference of 1950 largely corresponded to the pre-liberation "platform" of the CMA. In the one area in which the new guidelines deviated from the CMA's policy (Chung-i), actual policy was at variance with the normative guidelines of Chairman Mao.

The structure of the Wei-sheng-pu was no less important. The way in which the organization was built created constituencies and points of leverage which favored particular interests. For instance, Soviet medical experts had important roles in the Ministry. The fact that there was a dual emphasis on middle and higher medical education was a reflection of the same emphasis in the Russian system. Secondly, the traditional medical community had no institutional presence in the Wei-sheng-pu; its only governmental agency was in the Commerce Ministry. Thirdly, the health bureaus of the administrative regions were relatively autonomous, were dominated by physicians, and were political arenas in which leaders were relatively responsive to professional pressures. Finally, medical doctors dominated the Ministry's education and research bureaus. They quite predictably pushed for high quality work.

No less important was the fact that the Ministry's budget was small and the tasks enormous. Consequently, each subordinate administrative unit was given substantial tasks and had to find its own way to finance programs. This meant that large and prosperous urban areas had the greatest capacity to implement programs. Reinforcing the urban focus in curative services were several other factors: (1) National economic plans designated heavy industry as the top priority and the health system was supposed to be supportive of that effort. (2) The sudden coverage of Party and government cadres, along with millions of workers, meant that the politically and economically potent sectors of the society created an immediate demand for curative services; this effective demand was concentrated in the cities.

In sum, the institutional weakness of the Party gave the Ministry room for independence. In this political arena, medical professionals dominated. Policy, however, reflected not only these pressures but also objective economic constraints, foreign influence, and the role which the drive toward heavy industrialization imposed upon the Wei-sheng-pu. In the years to come, changes in developmental plans, Party strength, and the relationship with the Soviet Union could not help but find reflection in health policies. This is the story to which we now begin to turn.

NOTES

1. Ezra Vogel, Canton Under Communism (Cambridge: Harvard University Press, 1969), pp. 46-48.

2. Ezra Vogel, Interview No. 42. I would like to thank Professor Vogel for making available his extensive interview protocols with refugee physicians. For a table of Ministry organization see Appendix A.

3. Tai Cheng-hua, "Chung-kuo Jen-min Chieh-fang-chün Tsai Ti Erh T'se Kuo-nei Ko-ming Chan-cheng Shih-ch'i Te Wei-sheng Kung-tso Tsu-chih Ch'ing-k'uang" [The situation of the health organization of the Chinese People's Liberation Army during the period of the Second Revolutionary Civil War], I-hsüeh Shih Yü Pao-chien Tsu-chih [The history of medicine and health organization], no. 1 (1958), p. 34.

4. Agnes Smedley, The Great Road (New York: Monthly Review Press, 1956), p. 262; also, Donald W. Klein and Anne B. Clark, Biographic Dictionary of Chinese Communism (Cambridge: Harvard University Press, 1971), p. 286.

5. Who's Who in Communist China (Hong Kong: Union Research Institute, 1970), pp. 576-577.

6. Klein and Clark, p. 185.

7. David M. Lampton, Interview File 21 E, no. 5. This interviewee asserted that Tsui's move to Peking (despite being attacked in People's Daily) was a result of his close ties to Ch'en I.

8. Who's Who in Communist China, p. 232.

9. David M. Lampton, Interview File 21 C.

10. Franz Schurmann, Ideology and Organization in Communist China (Berkeley: University of California Press, 1966), p. 190.

11. Mao Tse-tung, "Instruction Concerning Examination of Leadership Work of Health Departments of Military Committees," Hsin Jen Wei [New people's health] (Peking: People's Health Press, 1967), pp. 6-7.

12. Michel Oksenberg, unpublished chronology: see also, Kenneth Lieberthal, A Research Guide to Central Party and Government Meetings in China: 1949-1975 (White Plains, New York: International Arts and Sciences Press, 1976), p. 61.

13. Mao Tse-tung, "Speech Made by Chairman Mao at a Standing Committee Meeting of the Central Committee," Hsin Jen Wei, p. 9; see also, Lieberthal, pp. 62-63.

14. These figures may be misleading because health expenditures of an unknown magnitude are carried in the national budget under other headings such as "economic construction" (ching-chi chien-she). See Chung-yang Ts'ai-cheng Fa-kuei Hui-pien [Compendium of central financial regulations] (Peking: Ts'ai cheng Ch'u-pan-she, 1957), p. 61.

15. Kuo Mo-jo, "Cultural and Educational Work During the Past Year," New China News Agency (hereafter NCNA), September 30, 1950, Current Background (hereafter CB), no. 15, pp. 2-3.

16. Hu Ch'uan-k'uei, "Medical Conditions in the Northwest," Ta-kung Pao [Impartial daily], August 8-9, 1951, CB, no. 109, p. 1-3.

17. Audrey Donnithorne, China's Economic System (New York: Praeger, 1967), p. 213; see also, Joyce Kallgren, "Social Welfare and China's Industrial Workers," in Chinese Communist Politics in Action, ed., A. Doak Barnett (Seattle: University of Washington Press, 1969), pp. 540-573.

18. Ezra Vogel, Interview No. 5.

19. "Pa Chu-i Chiu-cheng-kai Hsien Wei-sheng-yüan Kung-tso Jen-yüan Te Ts'o-wu" [Pay attention to

rectifying the errors of the employees of the county health departments], Ta-kung Pao [Impartial daily], June 20, 1952.

20. "Wei-sheng Chi-kuan Ying-kai Chu-i Kuan-li" [Health organizations ought to pay attention to management], Nan-fang Jih-pao [Southern daily], December 24, 1953.

21. Nai-ruenn Chen, Chinese Economic Statistics (Chicago: Aldine, 1967), p. 446.

22. As a percentage of the total central budget, the Ministry's share rose from 1 percent in 1950 to 2.6 percent in 1953. However, in 1953 the budgetary item "health" was expanded to include hsiang (townships) and ch'en. Also, the impact of free medical care was being felt. See, Chung-yang Ts'ai-cheng Fa-kuei Hui-pien [Compendium of central financial regulations] (Peking: Ts'ai-cheng Ch'u-pan-she, 1957).

23. "Private Physicians Form Joint Clinics," Chieh-fang Jih-pao [Liberation daily], November 14, 1951, in Survey of the China Mainland Press (hereafter SCMP), no. 229, p. 22.

24. "Association News," Chinese Medical Journal (hereafter CMJ) 67 (1949):403.

25. Fu Lien-chang, "Learn From the Advanced Soviet Medical Science with Resolution and Persistence," CMJ 75 (1957):870; see also, Su Ching-kuan, "What Are the Important Tasks for 1953?", Kuang-ming Jih-pao [Bright daily], January 29, 1953.

26. "Jen-min Wei-sheng Kung-tso Te Cheng-ch'üeh Fang-hsiang" [The correct direction in people's health work], Hsin-hua Yüeh-pao [New China monthly], November 1950, p. 166.

27. William Y. Chen, "Medicine and Public Health," China Quarterly (hereafter CQ), no. 6 (1961), p. 154.

28. Li Teh-ch'uan, "Report on Public Health," Jen-min Jih-pao [People's daily], October 31, 1951.

29. "Education and Health Work in 1953 Plans," NCNA, February 9, 1953, in SCMP, no. 511, p. 6.

30.   "Association News," CMJ 67 (1949):399-403; see also, "New Medical Education System Shows Results," People's Daily, November 3, 1951, in SCMP, no. 225, p. 19.

31.   "Association News," CMJ 69 (1951):449.

32.   Chiang Yi-hung, "The China Union Medical College," Ta-kung Pao [Impartial daily], June 27, 1951, in SCMP, no. 153, p. 28.

33.   "Chung-yang Jen-min Cheng-fu Wei-sheng-pu Fa-pu Chin-nien I Cheng Kung-tso Chih-shih" [The Central People's Government Ministry of Public Health issues year's health directives], Jen-min Jih-pao [People's daily], April 19, 1950.

34.   Ezra Vogel, Interview No. 42, p. 8.

35.   "Association News," CMJ 69 (1951):449.

36.   Cited in Richard P. Suttmeier, "Party Views of Science: The Record from the First Decade," CQ, no. 44 (1970), p. 151.

37.   "Association News," CMJ 69 (1951):450.

38.   "China Union Medical College Expands," NCNA, December 17, 1954.

39.   Ezra Vogel, Interview No. 42, p. 14.

40.   David M. Lampton, Interview Files 21 E and 21 H.

41.   "Chia-ch'iang Tang Tui Wei-sheng Kung-tso Te Ling-tao" [Strengthen the Party's leadership over health work], Jen-min Jih-pao [People's daily], March 28, 1953.

42.   Kao Kang, "Consolidate National Defense, Develop the Economy," Tung-pei Jih-pao [Northeast daily], February 28, 1951; see also, "Official Report on the Carrying Out of the 1951 People's Economic Plans in the Northeast," CB, no. 177, p. 9.

43.   "Health Work in Canton," Nan-fang Jih-pao [Southern daily], July 27, 1951, in SCMP, no. 150, p. 26.

44.   By 1955, Peking had over five times the number of hospital beds it had in 1949. See, "More Medical

Facilities in Peking Area," NCNA, September 13,
1955, in SCMP, no. 1129, p. 38. In 1955, it was
announced that the first Five-Year Plan called for
having 71 percent of all hospital beds in major
cities. See, NCNA, August 16, 1955, CB, no. 358,
p. 21.

45. Donnithorne, p. 213.

46. "40 Percent of Private Medical Practitioners
in Tientsin Get Organized," NCNA, October 8, 1955,
SCMP, no. 1152, p. 12.

47. Michel Oksenberg, Interview File 63a, No. 2,
p. 1. This is an interview with a former staff
member of the Ministry of Finance. I would like to
thank Professor Oksenberg for making these protocols
available.

48. "Pa Chu-i Chiu-cheng-kai Hsien Wei-sheng-yüan
Kung-tso Jen-yüan Te Ts'o-wu" [Pay attention to
rectifying the errors of the employees of the county
health departments], Ta-kung Pao [Impartial daily],
June 20, 1952. This article noted that a county
health department had asked for a subsidy and then
protested when it was denied.

49. "Wei-sheng Chi-kuan Ying-kai Chu-i Kuan-li"
[Health organizations ought to pay attention to
management], Nan-fang Jih-pao [Southern daily],
December 24, 1953; see also, Ch'ang-chiang Jih-pao
[Yangtze river daily], July 19, 1950. One Canton
hospital reportedly bought a quantity of drugs for
1,200¥ and sold it for 4,000¥.

50. Michel Oksenberg, Interview File 63a. Also,
the media frequently called for reformation of the
local taxation system.

51. Ezra Vogel, Interview No. 19, p. 1.

52. David M. Lampton, Interview File 21 K.

53. Ch'ang-chiang Jih-pao [Yangtze river daily],
July 19, 1950.

54. For more on urban-rural gaps see, David M.
Lampton, "The Roots of Inequality in Education and
Health Services in China: A First Look at Five
Provinces" (Paper delivered at the 30th Inter-
national Congress of Human Sciences in Asia and

North Africa, Mexico City, Mexico, August 3-8, 1976).

55. Mao Tse-tung, "The United Front in Cultural Work," Mao Tse-tung Chi [The collected writings of Mao Tse-tung] (Tokyo: Ho Tien Wu Szu, 1971) 9: 133-137.

56. This call was made at the First National Health Conference in August 1950.

57. Mao Tse-tung, "Instructions Concerning Examination of Leadership Work of Health Departments of Military Committees," Hsin Jen Wei, pp. 6-7.

58. "Directive Concerning the Union and Mutual Learning of Medical Professions," Jen-min Jih-pao [People's daily], May 19, 1951.

59. "Pen-shih Hsien-hou Tsu-chih Szu-shih-szu Ko Lien-ho Chen-so" [This city preliminarily organized 414 united clinics], Hsin-wen Jih-pao [Daily news], October 11, 1953. This article noted that there were all traditional, all western-style, and mixed united clinics.

60. For a much more detailed look at this entire period's policy toward Chung-i see, Ralph Croizier, Traditional Medicine in Modern China (Cambridge: Harvard University Press, 1968), Chapter 8.

61. "Ministry of Public Health Sets Up National Examination Committee for Health Workers," NCNA, April 9, 1953, in SCMP, no. 548, p. 11.

Chapter 3
PARTY WINDS PREVAIL OVER
MINISTRY WINDS (1954-1957)

<u>INTRODUCTION</u>

This was a benchmark period for the Chinese
polity, generally, and the health system specifically. The years 1955 through 1957 capsulize the
ambivalences which have characterized the entire
communist period. The problem has been how to produce fundamental social change and simultaneously
obtain the cooperation of the professionals necessary to make any such effort successful. Mao's
call for an upsurge in the countryside,[1] the Draft
Plan for Agricultural Development, the drive to
nationalize remaining independent manufacturing
and commercial enterprises, and the abolition of
the administrative regions all signalled a new
fact; the Chinese Communist Party was less willing
to tolerate "autonomous" seats of authority than
had previously been the case. The 1955 purge of
Kao Kang of the Northeast Bureau of the Communist
Party and Jao Shu-shih of the East China Bureau for
building "independent kingdoms" was further indication of this. The health system could not isolate
itself from these trends and the policies designed
to redress these imbalances.

As a consequence of increasing central Party
assertiveness, the Ministry's leadership underwent
some modifications and new institutions were created;
new voices were afforded influence. Policy responded to these changes. The enabling condition
for this increased Party role was central solidarity
and an increase in the Party's capabilities.[2]

Three problems were of special concern to Party
leaders, especially Mao: (1) Ministry leadership,
at all levels, was largely in the hands of medical
professionals who were resistant to political control. (2) The policy of "union and reform" of
traditional Chinese medicine had been implemented
with substantially more emphasis being placed on

45

"reform" than "union." (3) Costs within the
medical system were rising rapidly as a result of
the initiation of free and insured medical care and
rising urban incomes.[3] Some of these difficulties,
like costs, were only marginally within the Wei-
sheng-pu's control, but this was not the issue.
Central Party leadership and the diminution of
professional authority was the point of contention.

CHANGES IN LEADERSHIP

Leadership theory is central to the Chinese
Communists' understanding of administration. When
problems arose in the Wei-sheng-pu, they were not
viewed as the natural result of insufficient
resources, conflicting visions of the public good,
and the division of authority in complex organizations. They were seen as manifestations of leadership error. For Mao, as for Confucius, the virtuous
leader was recognized by the success of his policies.[4] The Ministry's major defect, from the Party
Center's perspective, was being "divorced from
Party leadership." "The most important [problem] is
that numerous health departments to varying degrees
have come under the influence of bourgeois thinking
and disregard political leadership."[5]
As early as 1953, the first rumblings against
the dominance of medical professionals in the
policy-making system could be heard. In March of
that year, the head of the East China Region's
Health Department, Tsui I-t'ien, was attacked for
resisting Party influence and being excessively
responsive to professional demands.[6] The following
month, Chairman Mao delivered a blistering attack
against the Wei-sheng-pu saying, "Then the fact exists
that there is no leadership, no politics, and no
serious administration of the business departments
[of the Ministry]."[7] Again in October, Mao attacked
the Ministry of Public Health at a Politburo meeting
for failing to exercise leadership over doctors.[8]
In November 1952, the former deputy secretary
of Kweichow Province, Hsu Yun-pei, was appointed
vice-minister of health. Until 1954, however, Hsu
remained the most junior vice-minister. His ascend-
ency within the Ministry had to await the removal
of the first vice-minister, Dr. Ho Ch'eng. Hsu, a
man with no medical experience, was brought into
the Ministry in order to lay the foundation for
more extensive Party control.[9]

In July 1954, Mao escalated the attacks by saying,

> The health departments not only failed to implement the Central Committee's directives concerning integration of traditional Chinese and western medicine, but also failed to solve the problem of unity between doctors of western medicine and doctors of traditional Chinese medicine . . . a health administrative department shall be abolished if it fails to do these tasks successfully. [10]

In the wake of this criticism, another vice-minister of health, Chang Kai, was appointed. Chang had been deputy director of the Third Field Army's Political Department.

Along with these appointees, who were supposed to bring the Ministry under tighter rein, two former heads of regional health departments acquired vice-ministerial portfolios: Dr. Ho Piao and Dr. Tsui I-t'ien. To what extent their elevation was an attempt by Ministry professionals to dilute the impact of the political appointees, and to what extent their promotion merely represented the need to absorb regional leaders who had been displaced by elimination of the regions, is uncertain.

Attacks on the Wei-sheng-pu reached a new intensity in May 1955, with the denunciation of Wang Pin, head of the Northeast Public Health Bureau. Wang's transgression? Opposition to traditional medicine.[11] Wang had written that "certain governmental and economic foundations produce certain medical health organization forms."[12] This was a delicate way of saying that feudal political and economic systems produce feudal medical systems. The fact that Wang headed the already mentioned National Examination Committee for Health Workers only sealed the indictment in his case.

The Party Center (Chung-yang), however, had still bigger fish to fry. On November 19, 1955, People's Daily carried a "confession" by First Vice-Minister Ho Ch'eng in which he admitted having opposed Chung-i. All his deviations, Ho asserted, derived from one source; "I was divorced from Party leadership."[13] Ho, it will be remembered, had led health work since the early 1930s. Following Ho's political passing, Wu Yun-fu, "a senior figure in Party discipline and inspection work," was appointed a vice-minister of public health, and Hsu Yun-pei became the prima figure in the Wei-sheng-pu. By

1956, the influence of medical professionals within the Ministry had been diluted, but by no means eliminated.

In explaining policy change, alteration of organizations assumes as much importance as alteration of leadership. In 1955, bureaus (chü) were designated offices (szu). The significance of this move was considerably more than semantic. A bureau could independently contact subordinate units while offices had to route external communications through the Administration Department (Ban-kung-t'ing).[14] The Administration Department was completely dominated by Party political cadres.

The second, and soon to be most important, institutional change was the removal of specific tasks from the Wei-sheng-pu's authority. New, and independent, structures were established. In November 1955, the Party Central Committee created the Nine Man Sub-committee on Schistosomiasis with prominent politicians such as K'o Ch'ing-shih and Wei Wen-po of Shanghai in leadership positions. The policies of the Sub-committee were implemented by Party committees at the provincial and county levels. In turn, local Party committees called ad hoc meetings in which antiparasite programs were formulated and recommendations for national policy made. This was a policy-making system in which medical professionals played little role. Doctors lost their capacity to substantially influence antiparasite policy.

As one would expect, the Ministry reacted negatively to this diminution of its authority. Minister of Public Health Li Teh-ch'uan cautioned for the need to temper the enthusiasm of the masses with the knowledge of medical professionals, especially in the area of cure and prevention of parasitic diseases.

> However, there have also been many defects in this work [schistosomiasis]. In some areas, there was a lack of the understanding of the stupendous and complicated nature of the task, and this gave rise to a feeling of hastiness or the inclination to belittle the enemy.[15]

Li's fears were well-founded, as we shall see later.

The last organizational change related to Chung-i, the cause celebre for the 1955-1956 purges.[16] Prior to 1957, the Bureau of Traditional Medicine (Chung-i-szu) had been in the Commerce Ministry. This institutional separation had made

48

the articulation of traditional medical interests
difficult. In order to rectify this, the Bureau of
Traditional Medicine was moved to the Wei-sheng-pu
in 1957. In China, as elsewhere, power significantly resides in position, and political actors know
this.

In sum, the Party used conventional bureaucratic strategies to increase the responsiveness of the
health policy-making system. Besides trying to
place reliable individuals in strategic positions,
organizational patterns within the Ministry changed.
Bureaus lost some of their independent authority and
traditional medical perspectives were institutionalized within the Wei-sheng-pu. Finally, in those
policy areas in which the Ministry of Public Health
had not moved with sufficient dispatch (antiparasite work), entirely new organizations were established. All of these moves had the impact of
widening the number of constituencies considered in
policy-making.

LEADERSHIP'S EVALUATION OF THE PROBLEMS

While it was possible to decree changes in
leadership and organizational structure, the health
problems faced were less tractable. In grappling
with these difficulties, the new leadership became
ensnared in the day-to-day administrative imperatives which had constrained its predecessors. Also,
the leadership was influenced by the large corps of
bureaucrats who continued in their jobs; already
there seemed to be a pervasive organizational perspective. The result? While policy changed, there
was substantial continuity with the pre-1955 phase.

The first problem facing the Ministry's leadership was, how could the organization's various
departments be staffed with politically reliable
and competent individuals? It was a difficulty akin
to the one an American president-elect faces when
he must choose high-level staffers and advisors for
policy areas about which he knows little or nothing.
At first, the new Ministry leadership emphasized
recruiting politically reliable cadres, hoping that
they would be able to acquire the requisite skills
to make supervision meaningful. Rapidly, however,
it became apparent that many of these cadres lacked
the educational background to acquire technical
skills. Consequently, by 1956 doctors were being
given Party membership in the hope of utilizing
their skills and transforming their ideology within

49

the Party. This expansion of Party ranks was occurring generally, and reflected the need for leadership in the rural areas, as well. The question soon arose, who was supervising whom? Throughout the 1950s and 1960s, the Ministry's bureaus were generally staffed by medical doctors, many of whom were in the Party.

Costs, waste, and simple budgetary shortages have plagued bureaucrats in China as everywhere else. While revolutionary rhetoric has characterized periods of increased Party authority, the Chinese have generally emphasized balanced budgets and conservative fiscal policies. As the new leadership took over, it faced rapidly increasing expenses and very slowly increasing financial resources. Attempts to balance budgets and cut costs are inherently "conservative" tasks. By the very nature of the job to be done, the perspective of the leadership was almost predetermined.

Rapidly rising costs were the result of at least two factors: waste[17] and rapidly increasing urban populations.[18] Pharmaceutical waste and excessive hospitalization resulted from the implementation of free and insured (lao-pao chih-liao) medical care without adequate management. The problem of rising costs with the implementation of new insurance and free medical care programs seems to be a universal phenomenon; it has been studied in England, the United States, and Scandinavia. For instance, Shanghai's 1954 health budget exceeded estimates by 2.58 million ¥,[19] Shantung's was over by 290,000¥,[20] and Tsingtao's was over by 26,474¥ (in the first quarter of 1955).[21] The reason for these deficits? People tended to use drugs wastefully (a portion of which had to be imported at considerable expense) and "many persons stayed in the hospital for two or more years, and some have stayed four, five or even more years."[22] Unnecessary utilization and waste, in turn, produced shortages, crowded facilities, and generally declining levels of service. There were frequent demands that something be done about this. In short, the new Ministry leadership was confronted by demands for expanded service, on the one hand, and the need to reduce costs on the other.

Even the problem of traditional medicine, which the new leaders had been brought in to "solve," proved intractable. First of all, the average income of traditional practitioners was exceedingly low, being one fifth to one tenth that of western-style physicians.[23] To raise the average wage level

50

of 500,000 traditional practitioners, however, would
have required funds that quite simply were unavailable. To let their wages rise when ruralites had to
pay for services would be tantamount to reducing the
availability of medical care in rural areas still
further. Compounding the difficulties, as other
government agencies emphasized the expansion of
industrial and food crops, the acreage allotted to
growing medicinal herbs declined; the price of
traditional medical preparations rose dramatically.[24]
Once again, one sees that leadership in one organization is constrained by the activities of external
agencies, irrespective of its own policy predispositions.

The other area of difficulty which Chung-i
presented was "united clinics." While about 30,000
united clinics had been established, many of them
were in precarious financial straits.[25] Because
they were largely staffed by traditional practitioners, especially in rural areas, any increase in
charges meant that such facilities would be used
less frequently. The availability of rural medical
care would decline further. Consequently, clinics
frequently sought loans from the county branch of
the People's Bank. While not all of the calculations
involved are known, banks seemed to be reluctant to
loan money to clinics, especially those of question-
able viability. This was especially true because
there were so many other places where scarce money
could be invested.

The final problem confronting the health
leadership was the result of the previous emphasis
on cure in the cities and prevention in the countryside, within the context of pervasive scarcities.
In the drive to increase production, industrial
safety had not received sufficient attention. In
China, as in the Soviet Union and elsewhere, enterprise managers tended to resist the implementation
of safety programs which would, in the short-run,
reduce their capacity to achieve production targets.[26] In rural areas, united clinics had not
provided adequate (virtually any) curative health
care to the peasants. Both of these problems were
magnified as Mao began to articulate his desires
for expanded welfare for peasants and more emphasis
on prevention. The Chairman's concerns in this area
were only part of his larger concern with agricultural development and urban-rural equality.

In sum, the changes in Ministry leadership and
organization only marginally altered the situation.
Many of the most important problems were generated

far beyond the Wei-sheng-pu. Costs ran away because of rapid expansion of labor union and Party rolls. Traditional herbs were scarce because national directives (and local cadres) emphasized other crops. United clinics were not viable because of the economic scarcities in rural areas and the inability of central agencies to subsidize them. In a real sense, the problems set the agenda for the leaders, rather than vice versa.

LEADERSHIP RESOURCES AND ANTICIPATED RESISTANCES

While the very nature of the problems confronting the leadership set the agenda, the scarcity of resources and the anticipated resistances circumscribed the range of options open to policy-makers. The first, and most pervasive, resource constraint was the budget. The budget sets allocations for each agency at the national, provincial, and county levels; there are relatively few sources of revenue outside the budget, although such sources can be important in particular cases. Just examining how the Wei-sheng-pu has fared in the budgetary struggle gives one the impression that it did not fare particularly well. The 406 million ¥ budget of 1955 was significantly less than the 565 million ¥ of 1953.[27] While the categories covered under the "health" item in the budget may have changed, it is clear that the Ministry had a dearth of resources relative to the responsibilities it faced.

Another critical constraint had not been changed by the increased role of non-professional medical leadership; the availability and utilization of Soviet experts. Russian medical experts still occupied bureau-level positions in the Ministry of Public Health. Because the relationship with Moscow was still close, and advisors in the Ministry still influential, substantial departures from the Soviet model were not yet likely, though they were brewing, as many of Mao's recently obtained speeches indicate.[28]

Perhaps the crucial factor which limited the scope of change was that the Wei-sheng-pu, at almost all levels, was still dominated by medical doctors. By 1956, doctors were veritably streaming into the Communist Party. Recruitment procedures had been slackened to the point that doctors (and other highly sought-after individuals) could be made Party members in a mere 24 hours. This rapid expansion of the Party reflected the regime's country-wide

52

effort to mollify intellectuals in the wake of the Hu Feng campaign of 1955. As one interviewee noted,

> . . . in 1956 there was a real opening up of the Party to "higher intellectuals" and only the really top professional people were invited in. He gave the example of XXX, the vice head of XX Medical College. The Party informed the branch secretary of the school that the next morning's newspaper would carry a story of XXX being made a Party member and would they make him a member before that time. . . . This man joined the Party in 24 hours.[29]

While we are unable to trace the lines of influence, resultant medical policy seems to reflect the moderating influence of professionals.

In the face of these rigidities, the Ministry ended up focusing primarily on administrative remedies for its difficulties. One major capability which the Wei-sheng-pu thought it had was the ability to reduce costs and waste through administrative fiat and reorganization.

In an attempt to make the system more efficient, inspection teams were sent to lower levels, where they hoped to exert added financial control. Secondly, the leadership encouraged medical personnel to see more patients. The Ministry believed that doctors were not seeing the maximum number of patients. In 1956, one article noted that doctors in Canton had, on the average, only seen 7.5 patients per day in 1955. By 1956, the daily patient load per doctor was alleged to have risen to 18.5.[30] The underlying assumption of all these reform efforts was that there was unused capacity.

The final resource which the Wei-sheng-pu could try to tap was the potential of other organizations. Bluntly, the Ministry could attempt to transfer the costs of its programs to other agencies or, as the Ministry put it, have other agencies pick up their "fair" share of the burdens. Arguments about the distribution of burdens in industrial health and pharmaceutical work were particularly common, as we shall see.

Concluding this section, the Ministry leadership had objective problems and limited resources. The relatively inelastic resources (money, expertise, and politically reliable supervisory personnel) were the most important in determining the Wei-sheng-pu's capacity to depart from past patterns of policy. Consequently, even though leadership changes had occurred, the breadth of policy change was limited, being most visible with respect to traditional medicine, the one area where a policy change did not require a vast infusion of resources. In fact, it was the slight magnitude of change in this period that convinced Mao that the activation of alternate policy-making arenas was necessary in the Great Leap Forward. Before getting ahead of the story, however, the immediate task is to analyze how leadership, perceptual, and resource changes affected the content of specific health policies.

HEALTH CARE ACTION POLICIES, 1954-1957

Medical education policy changed very little during this period, although tensions and problems abounded beneath the surface. The reasons for the outward stability were several: First, Soviet advisors in the Bureau of Medical Education were prominent; the Soviet medical education system found its mirror image in China.[31] Secondly, most changes in the scope and pattern of medical training would require a massive commitment of money which was unavailable. No less importantly, as long as the Ministry concentrated on restoring urban hospitals and constructing county curative facilities, there was a tendency to place emphasis on training doctors who had the capacity to work independently in a relatively specialized setting. Finally, the medical profession opposed any reduction in "standards" for personnel.

In February 1954, the Party Central Committee's Culture and Education Department called for an increase in the number of intermediate-level health personnel.[32] While manpower figures are not particularly good, it is clear that substantial acceleration in the training of such personnel did not occur. Counterposed to the Party's call for an increase in the number of lower and middle-level medical personnel, prestigious physicians were calling for a doubling of the enrollment in full-length medical schools by 1957.[33] Budgetary inadequacies, Soviet influence, the limited resources of local governments, the needs of the hospital system, and professional pressures all inhibited rapid expansion of middle-level personnel.

Medical research received more emphasis during this period, reflecting the general trend toward encouraging intellectuals and in recognition of the fact that little was known about many of China's

54

most pressing diseases. Because the funds for the Chinese Academy of Medical Sciences (founded in late 1956) came, in substantial part, from the Chinese Academy of Sciences,[34] the level of funding of the Academy of Sciences was an important determinant of research capabilities, perhaps more important than the budget allocations to the Wei-sheng-pu. Kuo Mo-jo noted that scientific research expenditures (1956) would rise 227.17 percent over 1955.[35] Paradoxically, while Ministry resources appeared to have decreased, medical research, formally under the Ministry, prospered.

This explanation, however, still leaves unanswered the question, why did the resources allocated to research increase so dramatically, especially at a time when the health budget was under such constraints and the national budget was in deficit?[36] Kuo offered an explanation when he noted that the Twelve-Year Plan for Science and Technology had been drawn up by "an elite group of over 200 senior scientists." Comrade Kuo went on to say, "I wish to make particular mention of the great help given us by Soviet advisors and experts in China."[37] The Chinese Medical Association (CMA) was another institutional force behind medical research. The month after Kuo's speech, Fu Lien-chang, the president of the CMA, addressed the 10th General Conference of the Association saying, "This meeting is for 'marching forward in modern science.'"[38]

While there was diverse support for medical research, there were conflicts. Because doctors had several roles (clinician, researcher, and educator), conflict arose over the allocation of time among those duties. For instance, the Ministry of Higher Education and the Education Bureau in the Wei-sheng-pu wanted emphasis placed on teaching. The Chinese Academy of Sciences and the Ministry's Scientific Committee on Medical Sciences preferred a heavier emphasis on research. Conflict resulted, as Yang Hsiu-feng, the minister of higher education, noted.

> The Academy of Sciences and various departments are working together to draw up a 12-year scientific research plan. . . . Inevitably the question of transferring the high-standard teachers . . . to reinforce the scientific force in their departments will also be considered by the Academy and departments. But if the teaching force of the higher educational institutions, which is already very short, . . . is reduced, the force for fostering scientific

cadres and technical cadres will be weakened.
Taking a long-range view, this would be disadvantageous. . . . The "vacant spots" and weak
links in scientific research organs are in
general precisely the "vacant spots" and weak
links in higher education.[39]

This discussion of research demonstrates two
characteristics of the Chinese political system.
First, within organizations and between organizations, there are alternate views of the public good
which tend to parallel organizational interests.
In China, as elsewhere, it is not objectively
obvious what is "serving the people." This intraorganizational fragmentation also provides the basis
for complex interorganizational coalitions. Secondly, patterns of budgetary allocation can be different than lines of organizational responsibility.
Research prospered under the Ministry while education
was constrained; funding sources differed.
Policy regarding the structure of the health
care delivery system had two characteristics:
(1) It remained urban centered and (2) it tried to
cope with rapidly escalating costs. These two
policy dimensions were closely related.
The initial trend toward concentrating hospital
construction in urban areas persisted. However, as
higher-level agricultural producers' cooperatives
(APC's) were being formed (late 1955) as a result of
"the socialist upsurge in the countryside," there
was a burgeoning number of rural group practices.
By 1956, some counties were claiming to have APC
clinics in all cooperatives.[40] The APC clinics were
essentially "united clinics" which had become linked
in name (not financially) with a particular APC.
As such, they solved virtually none of the problems
with rural health care. These clinics still
required direct patient payments, they tended to be
insolvent, and they were the focus for traditional
practitioners rather than centers for the diffusion
of western medical knowledge. While the Ministry
did not resist the establishment of these centers,
it did not allocate resources to them. Instead, it
focused its attentions on county hospitals.
From the perspective of the Ministry, the best
way it could meet rural health needs was to build up
the county hospitals and then try to insure that
ruralites had access to them. This had, in fact,
been the policy of the Kuomintang government twenty
years before. In this effort, the Wei-sheng-pu
pushed county health administrators to keep

56

facilities open longer hours and provide services which ruralites could use. However, from the perspective of local administrators, this policy compounded their financial and administrative burdens. Such central demands led to requests for subsidies which the Ministry generally could not provide.

Several factors reinforced the Ministry's policy of concentrating resources in urban areas. First of all, increasing urban incomes, rising levels of insurance, and free medical care kept urban demand high. For instance, the number of workers and other employees receiving free medical care in 1953 was 5.5 million, rising to 6.6 million by 1957.[41] Also, because state and Party cadres were concentrated in urban areas (and were entitled to medical benefits), the most potent political groups were demanding medical services. Finally, labor leaders (e.g., Li Li-san) were pushing for expanded benefits,[42] and union health funds had substantial treasuries.[43] In short, the money and political muscle were all in the cities. This fact is reflected in the growth of the number of insured workers in some of the major cities. For instance, in 1955, Canton had 11,015 insured workers; in 1956 it had 64,000.[44]

No less importantly, the major financial problems which the Ministry faced originated in the cities. Urban areas had to be put in order before anyone (in the Ministry) could imagine expanding services to the rural areas. In the cities, industrial health work, referral from enterprises, and cost problems were interrelated. Lack of preventive work in the factories generated patients that the hospitals were obliged to treat. Excessive referral from enterprises created patient logjams in district hospitals, and aggravated the financial problems. A two-pronged attack was launched: (1) The Ministry took a lead in trying to get other organizations to institute industrial health and safety programs and (2) it promoted regulations which would tighten up the procedures for referral.

In 1955, a Commission on Industrial Hygiene was established, composed of one vice-minister of health, one representative from each of the seven industrial ministries, a representative of the Ministry of Labor, and a member of the All China Federation of Trade Unions.[45] The purpose of the Commission was to coordinate the action of various agencies in achieving better and safer working conditions. While data are not extensive, one

knowledgeable interviewee noted that such efforts
at coordination were fraught with difficulty. The
major problem was that enterprises and the industrial ministries were hesitant to engage in extensive safety programs that would either slow production or the rate of capital accumulation.[46]
Labor leaders lacked the institutional strength and
financial resources to force through the programs
themselves. The Ministry of Public Health didn't
have the resources. As a consequence, labor safety
was more easily proposed than achieved. Even in
the mid-1970s, the obvious dearth of industrial
safety strikes most visitors.

The other approach to dealing with excessive
demands on urban facilities was to make it mandatory
for workers to be screened before they could gain
admittance to municipal facilities. The organizational device used was the "sectional medical service." Only with the approval of factory health
personnel could an employee go to the local hospital
or outpatient clinic, on other than an emergency
basis. The main function of this system, from the
Ministry's perspective, was to reduce the burdens
being placed on municipal hospitals. As People's
Daily noted,

> . . . rational adjustments of medical service
> contracts and proper organization of the masses
> of the people have eased the congestion at the
> large hospitals . . .[47]

In sum, the structure of the medical system
and the distribution of health services reflected
basic resource inadequacies and the constellation
of political forces that had an interest in specific
patterns of distribution. Every level of the system
tried to maximize its assets and minimize its liabilities. The industrial ministries tended to balk
at implementing extensive safety programs and the
Wei-sheng-pu tried to encourage this. Local county
hospitals asked for subsidies while the Ministry
tried to get them to perform more functions. Finally, because those who were entitled to free and
insured care were largely in the cities, the political pressures they exerted, and the financial problems they created, further focused the attention of
bureaucrats on urban areas. All this was reinforced
by the central investment decisions which called for
supporting the industrialization effort.

Financial policy was linked with decisions in
all other facets of health policy. Because the

Ministry leadership had no authority to independently alter its financial resources, most Ministry financial policies were limited to promoting regulations designed to reduce waste and increase management efficiency. This inability to fundamentally alter its own financial position had three implications: First, the Ministry generally saw itself as being victimized by forces beyond its control. Secondly, efforts to reduce waste and increase efficiency, from the patient's viewpoint, appeared to be bureaucratic insensitivity. Finally, budgetary scarcities produced conflict within the health system.

While budgetary data are fragmentary and often only available for non-comparable years, a few major trends come through, especially for the years 1954-1956. In 1954, the Ministry was allocated 490 million ¥; this fell by 18 percent, in 1955, to 406 million ¥. By 1956 it had risen, once again, to 489 million ¥ (or up by 17 percent), giving a net decline in the health budget of less than 1 percent between 1954-1956.[48] While some of this fluctuation may have been due to changes in accounting methods, it is clear that the Wei-sheng-pu's overall resources were not expanding, and may well have been shrinking.

While the total level of health resources was either stable or declining, some areas of expenditure were cut while others rose. For instance, between 1954 and 1956, expenditures for construction of new facilities and subsidization of existent facilities declined by 23 percent.[49] Such substantial declines quite naturally gave rise to cries of anguish from health facility administrators. While general support for subsidization was declining, expenditures for health in China's two major cities, Shanghai and Peking, were rising rapidly. From 1955-1957, Shanghai's health expenditures rose more than 2.2 times.[50] From 1955-1956, Peking's allocations rose 16 percent.[51] In short, while the total pool of budgetary resources was shrinking (or, at best, barely holding constant) the expenditures in major cities were rising rapidly. This reflected the greater tax base of the major cities, the concentration of cadres entitled to free medical care, and the central investment decisions of the First Five-Year Plan. While we would like to know how all these variables interacted, the data are not available.

As noted above, the concentration of cadres entitled to free medical care in the cities was one

reason for increased urban expenditures. While the
overall level of health expenditures had held stable
at best, the costs of free (kung-fei) health care rose
by 1.5 percent between 1954 and 1956.[52] With the
expansion of the Party in 1956-1957, the costs no
doubt soared, but we just do not know by how much.

Several trends stand out from these data.
First, the cities were where the budgets were
rapidly growing and it was in the cities that the
financial problems had to be solved first. Secondly,
probable declines in resources led to a lowering of
the capacity to subsidize institutions; this was
particularly detrimental to facilities in areas
outside of the major cities (e.g., county hospitals).
Finally, the costs of free health care appeared
stuck at high levels. In short, the Ministry's
primary financial concerns during this period were
increasing efficiency, and decreasing waste, primarily in the urban system.

Given the Ministry's inability to maintain high
levels of subsidization, the Wei-sheng-pu and local
health administrators tried to induce outside
agencies to supply the resources they were unable
to muster. The first rural financial problem which
caught the Wei-sheng-pu's attention was the plight
of "united clinics." The Ministry's internal news-
letter, Chien-k'ang Pao [Health bulletin] noted that
finances were "the biggest obstacle to the consolidation and development of united clinics."[53] In an
attempt to increase their viability, without adding
to central burdens, the Wei-sheng-pu asked the
county branches of the People's Bank to increase
the availability of loans.[54] The efficacy of this
request is unknown. Simultaneously, the Ministry
established "united clinic management areas" which
were supposed to boost efficiency in management and
procurement of supplies.

The most direct example of the health system's
attempts to get other agencies to absorb some costs
was evidenced when the head of a Provincial Health
Department requested the Commercial Ministry to
lower the price of drugs. ". . . if the Commercial
Ministry can qualitatively and quantitatively help,
by giving the hsien [county] aid, this would solve
the Health Ministry's previous difficulty of capital
insufficiency and then [we] can make a Great Leap
Forward in the speed of development of medical
work. . . ."[55] The position of the Commercial (and
Chemical) Ministry was that drug prices should only
be lowered when supplies were up, demand could be
met, and costs of production reduced.[56]

Within the urban system, the object was efficiency and the vehicle was "united management." The
idea of united management was to consolidate the
administration of several medical facilities and
thereby reduce costs. The simultaneous administration of several health facilities would reduce dupli-
cations in equipment and alleviate the need to maintain duplicate inventories. In addition, united
management was supposed to make it possible to
increase the utilization of hospital and sanatoria
beds. One article noted that there was only a 70
percent utilization rate for sanatoria beds.[57]

Finally, efforts to reduce cadre drug waste and
to diminish the number of unnecessary referrals to
municipal hospitals continued. While we have little
specific budget information, it is clear from the
increase in free medical care expenditures and the
increase in urban health budgets that these attempts
were not fully effective.

In sum, financial problems did not change as a
result of the new Ministry leadership. Because the
Ministry leadership could not unilaterally alter the
taxation and budgetary system, it was forced to try
and make the best use of available resources. By
the very situation in which it was embedded, efficiency became one of the few means by which the
leadership could cope with the economic constraints.
This meant that the provision of services had to be
more tightly controlled by administrative procedures.
By their very nature, these regulations alienated
"the masses" and the medical professionals in the
system.

Because resources were so limited, the Ministry
had to try and induce other agencies to provide
services which would help it meet its obligations.
The drug manufacturers, the People's Bank, and
industrial enterprises all tended to resist the
imposition of "peripheral" burdens on them. In
short, while we don't know all of the intricacies,
it is clear that a sophisticated game was being
played in which each agency tried to increase its
assets and reduce its burdens. Until the urban
system was put in order and resources increased,
the Ministry was in no position to expand the scope
of curative services provided ruralites and residents of small urban areas.

The conditions of physician employment began to
alter during this period. One of the major problems
which the Party leadership faced was the dilemma of
either staffing departments with politically reliable incompetents or politically dubious experts.

61

By 1956, the policy had definitely become one of making maximum use of doctors by recruiting them into the Chinese Communist Party. People's Daily noted,

> . . . the active development of education on communism among intellectuals, and the enlistment of Party members has become a problem which calls for urgent solution.[58]

While this liberalization was part of a national trend to be discussed in the following chapter, doctors were prominent among the persons being given Party status.[59] While we cannot specify the chain of influence, it is significant that the political content of medical curricula declined in 1956.[60]

Of all the trends we have noted, the decision to bring expertise into the Party was most significant for the future. Once doctors (and other professionals) were given Party status, the very homogeneity of organizational and political values was diluted. It was one thing for the Party to have control and it was quite another to figure out what the Party was (in operational and ideological terms) and which Party members were to exercise power. The incipient professionalization of the Party stems from the need to administer a complex society which produced problems such as those described above.

While doctors were playing a substantial role in medical institutions at all levels, and were joining the Party, they still had grievances which would have visible repercussions in the next period, as we shall see. Western-style doctors, in general, felt that research had been short-changed and that clinical demands were too onerous. At one meeting in 1956, for instance, "All present at the forum also criticized the negligence of the Ministry of Public Health in its leadership of scientific research."[61] Doctors had been alienated by increasing demands that they see more patients and work longer hours.

Policy vis à vis Chung-i changed most substantially. The emphasis on traditional medicine represented the combined result of the need to use all available medical resources, Mao's idiosyncratic interest in Chinese medicine, and the Party's desire to increase its control over independent professional and ministerial power. As Chairman Mao noted,

> Doctors of traditional Chinese medicine play a very significant role in the health of the

people, but this fact is seldom reflected to the leadership because doctors of traditional Chinese medicine are out of power while doctors of western medicine are in power.[62]

The question of power was at the heart of this controversy (and purge) in the Ministry. Mao had called for the integration of traditional and western-style medicine at least four times since 1949. In a People's Daily article blasting Vice-Minister Ho Ch'eng, Dr. Ho was accused of saying, "Health work is a special scientific and technical task. The Party does not understand scientific technique and therefore is incapable of providing leadership in this task."[63] Furthermore, the Wei-sheng-pu had defied explicit Central Committee orders. As Mao noted in July 1954,

> [Chung-i] was despised and repudiated. (For example, examinations for doctors of Chinese medicine were held in which there were papers on physiology and pathology. Those who failed these examinations were not given diplomas. In addition, there were regulations prohibiting doctors of Chinese medicine from entering hospitals.) The directive of the Party Central Committee has not been carried out.[64]

With the alterations in Ministry leadership and the movement of the Bureau of Traditional Medicine to the Wei-sheng-pu, the institutional and leadership base for a change in policy had been created.

In late 1955, a Chinese Medicine Research Institute was established, along with an unknown number of traditional Chinese hospitals.[65] In addition, four (five-year) colleges of traditional medicine were founded: one each in Peking, Shanghai, Canton, and Ch'engtu.

From these early days a fundamental ambiguity in policy was apparent. On the one hand, the new policy sought to provide traditional practitioners with a strong institutional base from which to operate and, on the other, it sought to bring about a "union" of the two traditions. In short, there were really two approaches: the "separate but equal" and the "total integration" paths. These two approaches were contradictory to the extent that creating an independent institutional base for Chung-i was an obstacle to the later fusion of the two traditions. As we shall see, the increasing strength of the traditional medical establishment gave coherence to another constituency opposed to total integration.

Policy toward mass campaigns reflected Mao's changing assessment of the potential of the peasants, the fact that hospitals were overcrowded, the changing patterns of disease, and basic issues of institutional power.

By 1954, many of the previously prevalent epidemic diseases had been brought under control, leaving the medical system with a more complex range of health problems demanding solution. In rural areas, parasitic diseases were built into the very fabric of agriculture. Millions of persons demanded cure, prevention was a massive undertaking, and there were often no widely accepted modes of prevention and/or treatment that were within the capabilities of the system. Schistosomiasis, a parasitic fluke disease, affected at least ten million persons in the Yangtze River Basin. This problem became the first focal point for antiparasite programs.

The Wei-sheng-pu's antischistosomiasis program had emphasized the need for basic research before implementing programs.

> Inadequate clinical, preventive and epidemiological knowledge concerning schistosomiasis
> . . . has greatly handicapped our fight against this disease. Therefore researches on schistosomiasis have been emphasized. . . . This work in the past few years has been carried out under the direct leadership of the Ministry of Health. . . .[66]

Professionals within the Ministry believed that treatment of the disease should only be carried out in properly equipped facilities using drugs and procedures which had been exhaustively tested.[67] Doctors were particularly worried about the unsupervised use of antimony drugs in the treatment of schistosomiasis because of their toxicity.

In contrast to the Ministry, the Party Central Committee was increasingly concerned about the need to bring about fundamental changes in the rural areas, and was aware that the Ministry program offered no immediate prospect of producing such alterations. Consequently, the Central Committee did what administrators often do; it set up an independent task force (the Nine Man Sub-committee on Schistosomiasis) to run the antischistosomiasis campaign. By 1956, the Sub-committee claimed to have trained 84,000 health workers and to have

64

treated 400,000 patients; plans were drawn up to
treat 1.2 million in 1957.[68]

The reasons that this campaign began when it
did are complex. First, basic power issues were
involved; the creation of the Sub-committee occurred
amid a general reduction in independent ministerial
authority and a purge of the Wei-sheng-pu. Secondly,
those placed in charge of the campaign (K'o Ch'ing-
shih, Wei Wen-po, and local Party Committees in
infected areas) were non-medical persons with the
greatest immediate interest in eradicating the
disease. In addition, hospitals in Shanghai (and
other urban areas) were being clogged with peasants
from outlying areas demanding treatment. Something
had to be done.

In the face of these pressures, only a few
options were open. The Ministry favored admitting
fewer patients and giving them longer, but relatively
safer, treatment. This implied either higher levels
of funding (which we have seen was very difficult
given the constraints of 1955 and 1956) or reducing
the number of individuals treated. The Party (outside the Ministry) believed that the best option
was prevention, mass treatment with potent drugs,
and reduced periods of hospitalization.[69]

The enabling condition for mass campaigns was
the increasing level of rural cooperativization.
Speaking of the period prior to the late 1955 drive
to establish cooperatives, one medical journal noted,

> . . . the fact that all the rural areas had not
> yet formed agricultural cooperatives prevented
> an overall program of prevention and treatment
> because there was no unified way of assigning
> the labor force or planning the use of the
> land.[70]

In short, the decision to establish the Nine
Man Sub-committee and launch mass antiparasite campaigns was the result of considerations which included rural needs and capabilities, changed disease
patterns, the desire to reduce professional power,
and the financial disabilities of the entire system.

SUMMARY

The common desire of Party leaders in Peking to
exert additional control over the Wei-sheng-pu produced leadership changes in the Ministry. This was
part of a larger effort to centralize control; the

purge of Kao Kang and Jao Shu-shih, along with the abolition of the administrative regions, was a reflection of this trend.

Once the new leadership was installed, policy change was most dramatic in those areas of highest salience to the new leaders and in those areas requiring the least expenditure of material and financial resources. Because policy toward Chung-i was of such high salience to Chairman Mao, and because the jobs of the new vice-ministers had been acquired largely over this issue, this area of policy changed most markedly. Such changes required relatively few central expenditures. While guide-lines toward Chung-i did change, these alterations would, themselves, become impediments to further union of traditional and western-style medicine. In creating an independent institutional structure for Chung-i, traditional doctors acquired an inter-est in not being swallowed up.

One of the central findings of this chapter has been that while some policy areas were "radicalized," not all were. Policy with regard to research is a good example. While a new institutional context was created for antiparasite programs (the Nine-Man Sub-committee on Schistosomiasis), a quite different political arena generated research policy. The Ministry's Scientific Committee on Medical Sciences, the Chinese Academy of Sciences, and the Chinese Academy of Medical Sciences were all bodies in which professionals and doctors had substantial influence. In the context of these committees and bureaus, the research budget witnessed a more than 200 percent increase (in 1956 alone).

Not only can different facets of health policy be moving in divergent directions, but also, many areas may not undergo change at all. This was the case in financial and educational policy. Educa-tional and financial guidelines were crucially dependent upon both the total quantity of economic resources and the administrative level at which they were controlled. Such basic decisions were made far beyond the Ministry. A dramatic move toward middle-level medical education could not be made until lower levels received the necessary resources. The capacity of the Ministry to provide such resources was diminished in this period. As we have seen, financial, educational, and delivery policy were all interlocking. When this fundamental cluster of issues was tackled in the next phase, political con-flict and bargaining were bound to occur. This is the story to which we now turn.

NOTES

1. Mao Tse-tung, "Selections From the Introductory Notes in the Socialist Upsurge in China's Countryside," Selected Readings From the Works of Mao Tse-tung (Peking: Foreign Languages Press, 1971), pp. 421-431.

2. John W. Lewis, Leadership in Communist China (Ithaca: Cornell University Press, 1963), pp. 108-120.

3. "Preliminary Directive on Free Medical Care for Those Involved in Building the Country At All Levels of the Government and the Party," Jen-min Jih-pao [People's daily], June 28, 1952.

4. Donald J. Munro, The Concept of Man in Early China (Stanford: Stanford University Press, 1973), Chapter 4.

5. Nan-fang Jih-pao [Southern daily], April 8, 1954.

6. "Chia-ch'iang Tang Tui Wei-sheng Kung-tso Te Ling-tao" [Strengthen Party leadership over health work], Jen-min Jih-pao [People's daily], March 28, 1953; see also, Kuang-ming Jih-pao [Bright daily], March 3, 1954. The latter article observed that all levels of the health system were "disregarding the Party."

7. Mao Tse-tung, "Instruction Concerning Examination of Leadership Work of Health Departments of Military Committees," Hsin Jen Wei [New people's health] (Peking: People's Health Press, 1967), p. 6.

8. Ch'üan-wu-ti [Invincible], no. 17, p. 2. An incomplete run of this Cultural Revolution tabloid is available in Hong Kong at the Union Research Institute. It is Red Guard document series no. 163.

9. David M. Lampton, Interview File 21 C.

10. "Secretary-General Ch'ien [Hsin-chung?] Relays Chairman Mao's Instructions on Traditional Chinese Medicine At Higher Medical Education Conference," Hsin Jen Wei, pp. 7-8.

11. "Openly Criticize Wang Pin's Bourgeois Thought of Discriminating Against Chinese Medicine," Nan-fang Jih-pao [Southern daily], May 19, 1955.

12. Jen-min Jih-pao [People's daily], December 28, 1954.

13. "Chien-ch'a Wo Tsai Wei-sheng Kung-tso-chung Te Ts'o-wu Ssu-hsiang" [Investigate my mistaken thinking on health work], Jen-min Jih-pao [People's daily], November 19, 1955.

14. David M. Lampton, Interview File 21 C.

15. Li Teh-ch'uan, "Speech to the 3rd Session of the First National People's Congress," Current Background (hereafter CB), no. 405, p. 12.

16. Li Teh-ch'uan, "Speech to the National People's Congress" (July 29, 1955), in CB, no. 351, pp. 25-32. Li laid out the ways in which Chung-i had been discriminated against.

17. "Kung-fei I-liao-chung Te Yan-chung Liang-fei Hsien-hsiang" [The phenomenon of serious waste in free medical care], Jen-min Jih-pao [People's daily], April 17, 1955.

18. Sun Kuang, "Urban Population Must be Controlled," Jen-min Jih-pao [People's daily], November 27, 1957, in Survey of the China Mainland Press (hereafter SCMP), no. 1668, pp. 3-7.

19. "The Phenomenon of Serious Waste in Free Medical Care." This was 16.7 percent over the budgeted amount. I would like to thank Nicholas Lardy for some of his budget data.

20. "The Phenomenon of Serious Waste in Free Medical Care." This was about 1.3 percent over the budgeted amount.

21. "Tsing-tao-shih Kung-fei I-liao-chung Liang-fei Hsien-hsiang Yan-chung," [The phenomenon of waste in free medical care in Tsingtao City is serious], Kuang-ming Jih-pao [Bright daily], June 22, 1955. This was 6.6 percent over the budgeted amount.

22. "The Hospital is not a Depository for Cadres," Jen-min Jih-pao [People's daily], May 1, 1955.

23. Kuang-chou Jih-pao [Canton daily], December 6, 1956. This article noted that the average traditional-style doctor received 30-40¥ each month and the average western-style physician received 150-300¥.

24. "Chia-ch'iang Tui Chung-yao Te Kuan-li Ho Yan-chiu Kung-tso" [Strengthen the management and research of Chinese drugs], Jen-min Jih-pao [People's daily], November 2, 1954. If 1950 were base year at price 100 (for Chinese drugs), then 1954's price level was 356.

25. Chien-k'ang Pao [Health bulletin], January 22, 1957; see also, "Chung-i Lien-ho Chen-so Yao Ch'iang Ling-tao" [Traditional Chinese united clinics must strengthen leadership], Nan-ching Jih-pao [Nanking daily], December 26, 1956.

26. "Jen-chen Tso-hao Kung-yeh Wei-sheng Kung-tso" [Conscientiously do a good job in industrial health work], Nan-fang Jih-pao [Southern daily], November 28, 1955; also, Mark G. Field, Soviet Socialized Medicine (New York: Free Press, 1967), pp. 101 and 103.

27. Nai-ruenn Chen, Chinese Economic Statistics (Chicago: Aldine, 1967), p. 446.

28. Mao Tse-tung, Mao Tse-tung Ssu-hsiang Wan-sui [Long live the thought of Mao Tse-tung] (Peking, 1969).

29. David M. Lampton, Interview File 21 E, no. 2, p. 3.

30. "Tang-ch'ien Wei-sheng Kung-tso Te Chi-ko Wen-t'i" [Several current problems in health work], Kuang-chou Jih-pao [Canton daily], December 7, 1956.

31. Ezra Vogel, Interview No. 42; see also, Victor Sidel, "Feldshers and Feldsherism in the Soviet Union," New England Journal of Medicine 278 (1968): 935-937.

32. Kuang-ming Jih-pao [Bright daily], March 3, 1954.

33. "Huang Chia-ssu Tai-piao Te Fa-yan" [Representative Huang Chia-ssu's speech], Ta-kung Pao [Impartial daily], August 1, 1955. Dr. Huang Chia-ssu made a call for more than doubling enrollments from 26,000 to 54,800. In fact, some of this occurred but our figures are inadequate to justify any precise statement.

34. Richard P. Suttmeier, "The Academy of Medical Sciences," in Medicine and Public Health in the

People's Republic of China, ed. Joseph R. Quinn
(Washington, D.C.: U.S. Department of Health,
Education, and Welfare, 1972), p. 178. Suttmeier
notes that the Chinese Academy of Medical Sciences
and the Academy of Agricultural Sciences "combined"
received 5-10 percent of the Academy of Sciences'
budget.

35. Kuo Mo-jo, "Development of Scientific Research
in China," New China News Agency (hereafter NCNA),
June 18, 1956, CB, no. 400, p. 1.

36. For a discussion of how to view the budget
deficit of 1956 see, "Tsai Yü-suan Ch'ih-tzu Wen-
t'i-shang Te Liang-chung Ken-pen Pu-t'ung Te T'ai-
tu" [Two basically different attitudes toward the
budget deficit], Chiao-hsüeh Yü Yen-chiu [Teaching
and research], no. 5 (1958), pp. 11-18.

37. Kuo Mo-jo, p. 2.

38. Fu Lien-chang, "General Conference of Chinese
Medical Association and Four Allied Societies,"
Chinese Medical Journal (hereafter CMJ) 74 (1956):
322.

39. Yang Hsiu-feng, "Higher Education in China,"
NCNA, June 20, 1956, CB, no. 400, p. 16.

40. "Wo-so K'an-tao Te Che-kiang-sheng San-ko
Hsien Te Nung-ts'un Wei-sheng Kung-tso" [My look at
health work in the villages of three counties in
Chekiang Province], Kuang-ming Jih-pao [Bright
daily], February 4, 1956.

41. Audrey Donnithorne, China's Economic System
(New York: Praeger, 1967), p. 213.

42. Paul Harper, "The Party and the Unions in
Communist China," China Quarterly (hereafter CQ),
no. 37 (1969), pp. 84-119.

43. CB, no. 382, p. 21 noted that labor insurance
funds in 1952 totalled 65.9 million ¥, 92.3 million
¥ in 1953, and 120 million ¥ in 1954.

44. David M. Lampton, "The Roots of Inequality in
Education and Health Services in China: A First
Look at Five Provinces" (Presented at the 30th
International Congress of Human Sciences in Asia and
North Africa, August 3-8, 1976, Mexico City, Mexico),
p. 35.

45. NCNA, February 25, 1955, in SCMP, no. 996, p. 4.

46. David M. Lampton, Interview File 21 K.

47. "Sectional Medical Service Adopted in Over Thirty Cities," Jen-min Jih-pao [People's daily], October 22, 1957, in SCMP, no. 1645, pp. 19-20; see also, Ezra Vogel, Interview No. 2, p. 1.

48. Disaggregated health budget data are available only through 1956. Also, the trends noted above would have been more stark if 1953 had been chosen as the base year; see, Nai-ruenn Chen, p. 446.

49. Feng Chi-hsi, "The Growth of the National Economy of China as Seen Through the State Budget," Ts'ai-cheng Kung-tso [Financial work], no. 12 (1957), pp. 28-33.

50. Nai-ruenn Chen, p. 450. There may be accounting explanations for some of this rise.

51. Nai-ruenn Chen, p. 449.

52. Feng Chi-hsi.

53. "Chin Hua Hsien Pang-chu Lien-ho Chen-so Chia-ch'iang Ts'ai-wu Kung-tso" [Chin Hua County helps united clinic strengthen its financial work], Chien-k'ang Pao [Health bulletin], January 22, 1957.

54. "Pang-chu Lien-ho Chen-so Chieh-chüeh Tang-ch'ien K'un-nan" [Help united clinics solve their present difficulties], Chien-k'ang Pao [Health bulletin], January 22, 1957.

55. Kwei-chow Jih-pao [Kweichow daily], July 29, 1956.

56. "More Medical Drugs for the Country," NCNA, March 13, 1956, in SCMP, no. 1249, p. 8.

57. Jen-min Jih-pao [People's daily], November 15, 1956.

58. "Make a Good Job of the Recruitment of Party Members Among Intellectuals," Jen-min Jih-pao [People's daily], March 21, 1956, in SCMP, no. 1259, p. 21.

59. "Higher Intellectuals Join the Chinese Communist Party in Different Parts of the Country,"

Jen-min Jih-pao [People's daily], March 12, 1956, in SCMP, no. 1259, p. 24.

60.   "Ministry of Public Health Holds Discussion Session to Revise Curricula of Higher Medical Institutions," NCNA, August 5, 1956, SCMP, no. 1356, p. 13.

61.   "Ministry of Public Health Holds Discussion," p. 14.

62.   "Speech Made by Chairman Mao at a Standing Committee Meeting of the Central Committee," (Spring 1955), Hsin Jen Wei, p. 9.

63.   "P'i-p'ing Ho Ch'eng T'ung-chih Tsai Tui-tai Chung-i Te Cheng-t'se-shang Te Ts'o-wu" [Criticize Comrade Ho Ch'eng's errors regarding the policy on treatment of traditional Chinese medicine], Jen-min Jih-pao [People's daily], November 20, 1955.

64.   Mao Tse-tung, "Tui Chung-i Kung-tso Te Chih-shih" [Directive regarding work on traditional Chinese medicine], in Mao Tse-tung Ssu-hsiang Wan-sui, pp. 10-11.

65.   Li Teh-ch'uan, "New Tasks for the Protection of Public Health," NCNA, June 1, 1956, CB, no. 405, p. 13.

66.   "Some Aspects of Research in the Prevention and Treatment of Schistosomiasis Japonica in New China," CMJ 73 (1955):101.

67.   "A Great Victory of Mao Tse-tung's Thought in the Battle Against Schistosomiasis," China's Medicine, no. 10 (1968), p. 594.

68.   Jen-min Jih-pao [People's daily], December 29, 1956.

69.   "A Great Victory of Mao Tse-tung's Thought," pp. 594-595.

70.   "A Great Victory of Mao Tse-tung's Thought," p. 592.

PART 2

LEADERSHIP AND ADMINISTRATION DIVIDED: THE GREAT LEAP FORWARD

Chapter 4
THE HUNDRED FLOWERS,
THE DIVISION OF ADMINISTRATION
AND THE ORIGINS
OF LEADERSHIP CONFLICT

INTRODUCTION

By 1957, the Chinese economic and political
system confronted a series of serious and interlocking difficulties. Agricultural production was
barely keeping up with population growth, slow
agricultural expansion was creating bottlenecks in
the industrial sector, extensive investment in the
cities and heavy industry had encouraged peasants
to migrate to urban areas in great numbers, and all
of these problems had helped generate hostility
toward the regime. No less importantly, strains in
the Sino-Soviet relationship were visible. These
tensions brought into question the degree to which
Peking could (or should) depend upon Moscow's
economic and military support and what the political
costs of such dependence might be.

In this context, a series of high-level conferences was held to reassess developmental policy.
This series began with the September to October 1957
Third Plenum of the Eighth Central Committee and
culminated with the August 1958 Peitaiho Conference
at which the Party Center approved a mass movement
to establish people's communes.[1] The Great Leap
Forward reached full speed. The Leap was an attempt
to rapidly accelerate agricultural growth and industrial production by concentrating rural resources
in larger (and presumably more efficient) production
units and by encouraging communes and localities to
construct their own small-scale industries. In
order to achieve both of these objectives, hundreds
of millions of people were mobilized. The leadership hoped to accomplish by sheer muscle and will-
power what had proven difficult to achieve through
a more measured developmental effort.

The health system could not remain insulated
from such a massive undertaking and, indeed, it had
an important role to play in the overall effort to

reduce urban-rural differences. Besides inadequate
resources, the major problem health policy-makers
faced during the Leap was that program authority
became divided among at least three political
arenas.[2] Each forum had little relationship to the
other, even though coordination of action was essential to the success of the overall program.[3]

This trend toward institutional division of
health policy-making responsibility had begun in
late 1955, with the establishment of the Nine Man
Sub-committee on Schistosomiasis. The further
division of authority during the Leap was merely an
acceleration of a previously existing trend; it was
not a complete break with the past. The critical
questions are: Why did additional fragmentation of
institutional authority occur at this time? What
identifiable consequences did this division of
responsibility have? To answer these questions, one
needs to examine the results of the Hundred Flowers
Campaign of 1956-1957 and look at the process by
which a reevaluation of the developmental strategy
occurred. In order to accomplish this, we shall
identify the major policy-making arenas, discuss
the critical participants, and analyze their perceptions of both the problems and the available
resources. Chapter 5 will deal with resultant
policy.

LEADERSHIP COMPOSITION

The prevailing wisdom concerning Party-govern-
ment relations during the Great Leap Forward was
summarized by Audrey Donnithorne. ". . . Party
organs came to overshadow the parallel government
bodies, and also to take over management of enterprises and other concerns."[4] This formulation gives
one the impression that there was only one identifiable seat of health policy-making authority and
that "the Party" (irrespective of issue and level)
was in firm control. This view is defective for at
least two reasons: (1) There were at least three
largely separate health policy-making arenas.
(2) The Party leaders of the Ministry of Public
Health, for instance, were a far different group of
persons than the Party leaders of the Nine Man Sub-
committee. In short, the Party was not a homogeneous organization.

The Nine Man Sub-committee, as noted above, had
been established in November 1955, under the direct
supervision of the Party Central Committee.[5] K'o

Ch'ing-shih, the Sub-committee's chairman, had had
a long Party career and had been named first secretary of the Shanghai Municipal Party Committee by
January 1955.[6] K'o was probably chosen for the Sub-
committee chairmanship for two reasons: (1) He was
a good organizer with strong ties to Mao and,
(2) Shanghai's ten suburban counties (along with the
entire Yangtze drainage basin) were most beset with
the schistosomiasis problem. In any case, K'o, a
man with no medical background, strong political
loyalties, and substantial organizational skills was
chosen to head mass antiparasite work in China.

The vice-chairman of the Sub-committee was Wei
Wen-po.[7] Wei, too, had been a Party loyalist,
having been a vice-minister of justice and secretary
of the Secretariat of the Shanghai Party Committee.[8]
Like K'o, Wei had no medical experience.

Another member of the Nine Man Sub-committee
was Liao Lu-yen, a vice-director of the Party's
Rural Work Department and minister of agriculture.[9]
Liao's primary concern was agricultural policy. It
was logical that something of as much impact upon
agriculture as mass antiparasite campaigns would
come under his purview. Liao, like his colleagues,
had no medical experience. The final publicly
announced appointment to the Sub-committee was that
of Hsu Yun-pei.[10] Hsu, as noted in the previous
chapter, had been brought into the Ministry of
Public Health in order to bring it under tighter
political rein.

In order to formulate antiparasite policy, the
Sub-committee held a series of ad hoc meetings. The
First National Antischistosomiasis Meeting was held
in November 1955, followed by a second in August
1956, a third in December of that year, a fourth in
February 1958, another in 1958, and a sixth in
1959.[11] At the 1956 meetings, Ministry of Public
Health and medical experts were much more conspicuous than in 1958, when specialists were accused of
being "sectarian" and "obstructionist."[12]

These ad hoc meetings were most responsive to
two kinds of inputs: agrarian demands that the
major parasitic diseases be brought under control
and the predilections of upwardly mobile cadres at
the commune, hsiang (township), and county levels
who promoted the movements. Mao described the
biases of such middle-level cadres, and the dangers
of listening to them.

> . . . we must not believe too much the state-
> ments made by such people as general branch

77

secretaries, secretaries of factories and
mines . . ., responsible persons of organizations under the municipal government and secretaries of Party groups. . . . Many of these
people have become almost completely divorced
from the masses. . . . On many issues they only
believe in themselves and do not trust the
masses. . . . The higher echelons and the basic
level will attack the middle level on both
flanks. Only by so doing can erroneous views
held by the middle-level cadres be recti-
fied. . . .[13]

In short, the Nine Man Sub-committee was subjected
to a different spectrum of pressures than the Wei-
sheng-pu . These were pressures that generated a
bias toward "campaigns of quick decision." Both K'o
and Wei had participated in the revolution dating
back to the 1920s and shared in the Party's mobilizational legacy. Also, the Sub-committee's leadership,
with no medical expertise, was in no position to
evaluate the claims of middle-level cadres. Finally, being politicians in Shanghai, they had a
stake in the rapid diminution of the parasitic
disease problem which was especially serious there.
    A bias toward mobilizational activity was not
only built into the Sub-committee policy-making
apparatus, it was also built into the implementation
structure. Party Committees at the county and above
levels were given responsibility for implementing
Sub-committee policies.[14] These Party Committees
had only minimal access to medical expertise and
were not arenas in which the restraining influence
of professionals was likely to be effective.
    In sum, the Nine Man Sub-committee was an arena
that had its own leadership, its own structural
characteristics, and its own capacities for action.
Quite naturally, policy coming from an arena such
as this would be substantially different than that
emerging from the Ministry of Public Health and the
communes.
    The communes, by the end of 1958, constituted
another policy-making forum. While there were significant differences between individual communes,
the range of pressures and political forces shaping
policy in them was similar. The decision to encourage the nationwide establishment of communes in
August 1958[15] created another type of arena in which
health policy (below the county level) would be made.
    Commune clinics in 1958 (unlike those of the
post-Cultural Revolution era) were almost wholly

independent of the Wei-sheng-pu. They were the
responsibility of Commune Party Committees. These
Party Committees were an historically unique type
of organization because of their extensive geographic coverage and the dominance of middle-level
cadres who had relatively tenuous links to both the
governmental apparatus and the local populace.
Donnithorne describes the motivations of much of
this commune leadership, and distinguishes it from
lower-level rural leadership (at the village level).

> It can be seen that a significant dividing line
> runs between those who are "state cadres" and
> who look to higher rungs of Party and state
> hierarchies for the approbation which can
> further their careers and the lower cadres who
> are first and foremost local peasants, subject
> to pressure from their fellows.[16]

Equally important, commune-level cadres were resistant to the influence of the governmental apparatus
(in this case the Wei-sheng-pu). In short, these
middle-level cadres in the enormous communes of 1958
were subject to very few restraining influences.

Amidst the zealotry of the Great Leap Forward,
and in the absence of professional and local linkages, there was a tendency for commune-level cadres
to immediately push programs which were highly
redistributive, even if local conditions might not
have been particularly favorable to such efforts.
Cadres perceived (probably correctly) that they were
evaluated on the basis of their performance in transforming rural areas, not on their facility for
articulating the "conservative" views of either
medical professionals or peasants. Because free
medical care was thought to be a tangible incentive
for higher levels of collectivization, it was one
of the first welfare functions initiated.[17] To
conclude, the communes and the Nine Man Sub-committee were both policy-making arenas in which the
capacity for policy innovation outstripped the
capacity or desire for taking professional and
local opinion into consideration.

The Wei-sheng-pu. While certain policy areas
were being handled by one or the other of the
aforementioned arenas, other responsibilities
remained within the purview of the Ministry of
Public Health. As a consequence, we must briefly
acknowledge the minor alterations in the Ministry's
leadership.

After the anti-rightist campaign of 1957-1958, some Ministry bureau heads were removed from their posts and replaced with younger Party physicians.[18] At the vice-ministerial level, however, no one was removed. In fact, one significant addition was made; Dr. Ch'ien Hsin-chung was appointed vice-minister of health in October 1957. Ch'ien had been the Southwestern Region's director of public health in the early 1950s and had been in the Soviet Union for advanced training in the mid-1950s. He was a great proponent of medical research.[19] While one should not make too much of one additional medical appointee (and several bureau-level changes), the role of medical professionals within the Ministry was certainly not diminished during the Leap and it may have been strengthened. One would anticipate that in those issues which remained under Wei-sheng-pu control (e.g., medical research, medical education, and hospital administration), the imprint of medical professionals would be much more apparent than in commune and antiparasite work.

THE LEADERSHIP'S DEFINITION OF THE SITUATION

Up to now, we have not fully discussed the Hundred Flowers Movement (of 1956-1957). This omission was intentional because this period can be viewed as a time in which various sectors of the Chinese society, bureaucracy, and political apparatus defined the major problems. In part, the differing policy prescriptions of the three policy arenas stemmed from divergences in basic perceptions about what the problems were.

Mao's definition of the situation. With qualifications that need not detain us at this point, essentially the same perceptions gave birth to the communes as led to a vast expansion in the activities of the Nine Man Sub-committee. Because both of these arenas became the vehicles by which a new rural vision was to be realized, the perceptual underpinnings of both arenas may be analyzed simultaneously. Mao confirms that there was a definite division of responsibility among the various arenas, with the Party leading the transformation and the government administering ongoing programs.

The major powers grasped by the Central Committee consist only of revolution and agriculture. The rest are in the hands of the State Council.[20]

80

Of course, the problem with this formulation was
that there was no way to disentangle the effort to
transform rural areas from the ongoing programs of
the bureaucracy.

As early as 1956, the Chairman began to realize
that the unbalanced economic development characteristic of the First Five-Year Plan was having an
adverse effect upon both the rate of growth and
political stability.[21] Additionally, lopsided
economic development was creating social inequalities (such as the urban-rural gap) which would be
increasingly difficult to rectify the longer the
process continued.

> . . . industry must develop together with
> agriculture, for only thus can industry secure
> raw materials and a market, and only thus is it
> possible to accumulate fairly large funds for
> building a powerful heavy industry. . . . As
> agriculture and light industry develop, heavy
> industry, assured of its markets and funds,
> will grow faster.[22]

In the Hundred Flowers Movement, the political
costs of the previous developmental strategy had
become apparent. After his insistence that Party
leaders (especially Liu Shao-ch'i and P'eng Chen)
permit public criticism of the Party, intellectuals,
workers, and peasants within and outside that organization blasted past policies from all directions. The
Chairman decided that both a basic change in developmental strategy and a new reliance on mass organizations was required. One of the most worrisome
problems to Mao was the apparent alienation of the
peasantry over a whole range of issues, one of which
was health care.[23] One broadcast noted, "The peasants feel that the Government is paying too much
attention to the cities. As a result, the workers
and cadres are leading a good life while the life
led by the peasants is a hard one."[24]

Additional problems resulted from the discrep-
ancy between urban and rural living standards.
Cities became magnets to peasants who sought to
improve their livelihood. In 1957 and 1958, the
deluge into the cities overloaded the basic social
welfare and maintenance institutions.

> The first result is the shortage of housing.
> . . . With the population of the cities growing,
> effects are produced on the supply of goods
> situation. . . . The larger the cities grow,
> the greater the expenditure of the state.[25]

81

In order to overcome both the inequalities, and
the concrete problems which resulted from them, the
Chairman felt that efforts had to be made to increase agricultural production and to raise the
level of services available to peasants; to, in his
words, consolidate the "peasant alliance."
Regarding the first point, Mao stated in his second
speech to the Second Session of the Eighth Central
Committee (May 17, 1958) that, ". . . the basic
problem is agriculture. . . ."[26] Regarding increasing the level of health services, the Chairman
had said several years before,

> . . . the scale and rate of the development of
> science, culture, education, public health, and
> so on, can no longer be entirely the same as
> originally intended. All must be appropriately
> expanded and accelerated. . . . Many of the
> diseases most harmful to man, such as schisto-
> somiasis, diseases formerly considered incur-
> able, we now are able to treat. In short,
> the people can see the great road open before
> them.[27]

Not only had previous policies deemphasized
rural welfare, they had also led to the creation of
intra-urban inequalities. No more than 25 percent
of China's city dwellers were entitled to free
medical care.[28] These inequities had produced disruptions during the Hundred Flowers Campaign.

> Some of the problems involving public mess
> halls, lavatories, medical clinics and dormi-
> tories which could and should be solved are
> left unsolved. In the case of those which
> cannot be solved, the reason is not made known
> to the workers. This is also a cause of dis-
> satisfaction among the workers. . . .[29]

By mid-1958, then, Mao had come to the view
that cost problems in the health system, economic
difficulties, poor performance in agriculture, and
political instabilities were all closely linked
together. The remedy had to be found in revitalizing
the agricultural sector. With the "intellectuals"
having proven unreliable, the chosen instrument was
to be mass organization, an approach perfectly consistent with the pre-liberation legacy of the base
areas. As well, however, the Chairman was prepared
to leave the Ministry substantial areas of responsibility. As a consequence, the perceptions of

Wei-sheng-pu bureaucrats were salient in determining policy outcomes in those areas under their
control.

The Wei-sheng-pu's perceptions of the problems.
The Ministry's leaders were fully aware that the
purges of 1955, along with the concomitant increase
in political penetration of the Ministry, had
resulted in hostility among medical professionals.
This hostility became conspicuous during the relaxation of 1956-1957. President C. U. Lee (of China
Union Medical College) had said, "The quality of
the work of Union College has deteriorated. . . .
The whole of Union College is in chaos; the Party
Committees are simply hopeless. . . ."[30] The head
of the Sian Academy of Sciences attacked the Party
for its antiresearch bias.[31] Nurses complained
that the Party had precipitated a decline in standards for nurses.[32] Succinctly, the first major
problem facing the Wei-sheng-pu's leadership was
disaffection within its own structure and in the
larger medical community.

Below this first-order problem, many difficulties required attention. While Mao's analysis
assumed that the central problem was undersupply
and underutilization of available resources, the
Ministry faced what it perceived to be excess
demand. Too many people were entitled to free or
insured medical care. As People's Daily pointed
out,

> . . . there must be revised certain existing
> measures which tend to encourage the rural
> population to infiltrate into the cities, such
> as subsidies for housing for workers, payment
> by the state of half the medical expenses for
> dependents of workers, and the additional issue
> of food and cloth ration coupons.[33]

The relatively high level of benefits in the cities
(along with increased opportunities for employment)
produced a rapidly expanding urban population. The
case of Kwangtung is illustrative; in excess of one
million persons moved to urban areas in that province in 1958 alone.[34] As a consequence of this
influx, conditions within medical facilities
deteriorated.

> Conditions deteriorated greatly during the
> years 1956 to 1961. Nurses' uniforms, once
> clean, were crumpled and dirty and gray, and
> bed sheets and pillows were not changed once
> during respondent's stay of over one week.[35]

83

The Ministry's assessment that it faced a situation of excess demand led it to initiate action which put it in a vulnerable political position. In the short-run, the only way to diminish costs was to reduce either quality of service or ease of access.[36] Either of these two alternatives was bound to alienate patients.

As we noted briefly in the preceding chapter, faced with excess demand, the Ministry has usually tried to increase management efficiency. Vice-Minister of Public Health Ho Piao said that too many hospitals wanted to "modernize" too rapidly and, in the process, they had purchased excessive amounts of expensive equipment.[37] Besides over capitalization of some facilities, drugs were being wasted and patients were permitted to stay in the hospitals for excessive periods.[38] Finally, cadres were abusing the privilege of free medical care. One Ministry report from Shanghai observed, ". . . according to statistics from Shanghai, the great majority of those receiving free medical care are young cadres, students and workers . . . each year they, on the average, visit a clinic 12 or 13 times."[39]

With the initiation of commune health centers in August 1958, an entire panorama of new problems confronted the Wei-sheng-pu. Each commune clinic was to have approximately one or two doctors per 2,000 population.[40] At this population-to-physician ratio, China needed between 300,000 and 600,000 doctors (not including those needed to staff urban facilities). Given the fact that there were only about 131,000 middle-level doctors, and only about 75,000 fully trained physicians,[41] it was impossible to satisfy the immediate demands for manpower which the communes were generating. Another problem which commune facilities created for the Wei-sheng-pu was that while they were not directly dependent upon the state budget, they competed with hospitals for drugs, personnel, and equipment. They aggravated the shortages which were already alienating doctors, urbanites, and those entitled to free medical care.

A final problem facing the Ministry of Public Health was, how could local health stations relate to the mass movements which the Nine Man Sub-committee was running? An internal Ministry document put the problem succinctly.

They [in the Ministry-run disease prevention stations] realize preventive health stations are technical departments. If they engage in patriotic health movement work, then this will weaken the strength of preventive health work.[42]

84

In conclusion, the Ministry leadership was presented with conflicting demands for better service
from the population while its financial resources
were being constricted and its burdens were becoming
more onerous. Every attempt it made to reduce
demand was bound to alienate some sector of the
population. In addition, as the communes and Sub-
committee moved into high gear, they created severe
problems of policy coordination and resource allocation with which the Wei-sheng-pu was unable to
cope. Finally, the leadership was constrained by
the dissatisfaction which the imposition of political
values created among the professionals within the
organization and the wider medical community. In
short, the Ministry's definition of the situation
meant that it would be less prone to embark upon
sharp policy departures than the other two policy-
making arenas.

LEADERSHIP RESOURCES

Mao's view of the available resources provided
the raison d'être for the Nine Man Sub-committee and
communes. In the absence of information about the
perceptions of leaders on the Sub-committee and in
the communes, we shall analyze Mao's appraisal of
the resource situation in the belief that his views
closely approximated those of leaders in the communes and on the Sub-committee. The Chairman
believed that great manpower resources remained
untapped and that the mobilization legacy of the
pre-1949 period was the key to their utilization.
As Mao remarked in March 1958 at the Ch'engtu Conference, the base area legacy had been forgotten in
the rush to emulate the Soviet Union.[43] Mao was
particularly concerned about the fact that the
Soviets seemed to be oblivious to the political
consequences of developmental programs; difficulties
had become most apparent in the criticisms leveled
against the Party in early 1957. As he said at the
April 1958 Hankow Conference, "We must not follow
the example of the Soviet academicians who give no
attention to the internal contradictions among the
people."[44] In the health field, the Chairman no
longer saw Moscow as a major resource in meeting
China's health problems. Shortly after Khrushchev's
1958 trip to the People's Republic, Wen-hui Pao
vocalized the new line.

What methods should we use for prevention?
There are two methods. One method is the

85

> excessive worship of documents, the excessive
> worship of the foreign, being divorced from
> production, and sitting and waiting for patients
> to come; this is the bourgeois method. The
> other method is believing in the creativity of
> the masses . . . this is the way of the working
> class.[45]

At the Ch'engtu Meeting, the Chairman recounted a
humorous anecdote that reinforced this perspective.

> After liberation economic and education work
> has given rise to dogmatism. . . . Health work
> is the same, and has harmed me in that for
> three years I could not eat duck eggs, and could
> not eat duck soup, because the Soviet Union had
> an article which says [one] could not eat duck
> eggs and duck soup, and then afterwards [the
> Soviets] once again said that [one] could eat
> them. It doesn't matter whether the articles
> are true or false, the Chinese all abide by it,
> all promote it. To sum up, the Soviet Union is
> number one.[46]

Much of the reason for the increase in mass
capabilities, in Mao's view, was the high level of
cooperativization that had been achieved. According
to Bernstein, by June 1956, about 90 percent of
China's peasants were either in higher or lower-
stage cooperatives.[47] By 1958, communes looked like
the next logical step for Mao; they were appealing
to him on several grounds related to health care.
First, peasants could be organized into work forces
to build capital improvements; this would have been
almost impossible under a system of private or
small-scale land ownership. Such a capacity was
particularly important in fighting parasitic
diseases.
     Besides providing the organizational prerequi-
sites for harnessing the energy of China's peasants,
communes were supposed to provide the finances for
extensive "free" medical and welfare activities. In
late 1957 and 1958, there was a series of upward re-
visions in the grain quotas based on reports of a
bumper harvest. Mao believed that the entire
resource picture of China was changing. With increasing abundance there was the opportunity to stem
the political alienation that he found so worrisome.
At the Hankow Meeting Mao said,

> After rectification last year, the bumper har-
> vest this year especially, and the (fundamental

86

or preliminary) transformation of our backward-
ness with three more years of hard struggle,
the people will understand and become convinced.[48]

Another resource which Mao believed was available was the Chinese people's acceptance of traditional medicine. While the Chairman's optimism
about the potential of Chung-i was greater than that
of many commune cadres (an important source of
friction as we shall see), he believed that the
therapeutic skills of Chinese medicine could be
learned rapidly in the context of mass campaigns.[49]
Growing medicinal herbs seemed like a low cost way
of increasing pharmaceutical availability; one merely
had to increase the acreage allotted to herb production. The attractiveness of this alternative,
however, proved overrated because communes had to
allocate their land to growing medicinal products;
many felt that the utility of growing food and
industrial crops was greater. The agricultural
stagnation of 1959-1960 just made the choice that
much starker. Even as early as late 1958, the
State Council noted that traditional drug production had reached only a third of its quota.[50]
In sum, the Chairman believed there were
three types of previously untapped resources:
(1) China's peasants were waiting to be harnessed
to transform the face of rural China. (2) Increased
rural health and welfare benefits could be financed
from increased agricultural production. This would
overcome the bottleneck which the central budget
represented. (3) Traditional medicine was "a great
treasurehouse" which held out the hope of rapidly
expanding the volume of pharmaceuticals and the
number of medical personnel. The leadership's capacity to tap these resources, however, was dependent
on at least three conditions: Agricultural production had to expand rapidly, peasant morale had to
be high enough to permit mobilization, and ruralites
had to be willing to use commune health personnel
rather than flooding urban hospitals. By 1960, all
three of these preconditions had ceased to exist.
The Wei-sheng-pu's appraisal of resources. As
we have repeatedly seen, the Wei-sheng-pu leadership
tended to rely on its capacity to increase system
efficiency. A revealing study appeared in 1958
which observed that each outpatient visit to a large
urban hospital cost 1.29¥, and per diem inpatient
costs were 4.59¥. By contrast, outpatient costs at
a county or district hospital were .94¥ and per diem

inpatient costs were 2.79¥.[51] The conclusion to which the Ministry came was that it was better to treat people at lower-level institutions. This demonstrates the basic attitude of the Ministry toward county hospitals. In choosing the level at which to concentrate curative care there is a trade-off between unit size (and costs) and the comprehensiveness of the services provided. For example, a larger unit provides more comprehensive care, but, the costs of rendering this higher quality care to a few patients increases the costs for all. Conversely, creating small commune clinics increases convenience and reduces costs, but provides less comprehensive service to those who may need it. In general, the Ministry has felt that the county is the optimal level in terms of the tradeoff between costs and comprehensiveness. As a consequence, the Wei-sheng-pu has concentrated its attention on increasing the capacity and convenience of facilities at this level. This does not mean that Mao opposed county hospitals. He did, however, favor creation of local curative centers which necessitated a diversion of resources away from the county hospitals and which increased their burdens.

Because the Ministry believed that one way to cope with cost problems was to increase the capacity of county and district hospitals, the financial underpinnings of facilities at this level were of the highest salience. In 1958, however, the national health budget declined by about 6 percent; this at a time when total national expenditures rose about 41 percent.[52] The conventional interpretation of this has been that the changes in the taxation system in 1958 increased the resources available to provincial and county units. The tax reform of 1958 did virtually eliminate tzu-ch'ou (self-help) taxes and did allocate a portion of surtax revenues to local units in their place.[53] However, it appears that there was little, if any, real increase in the total resources available to local units. Looking at provincial per capita expenditures for health, education and welfare during 1958, there is virtually no increase for the major provinces.[54] If one considers that provinces had greatly expanded responsibilities in 1958-1959, even the increased health budget of 1959 provided only marginal relief to harassed local health administrators. In short, the total pool of resources available to county and district hospitals certainly did not increase anywhere nearly as fast as the demands upon them. This meant that the Ministry was in its usual financial bind.

It had to increase the burdens of local units without being able to improve their financial position appreciably.

While the Ministry has never been conspicuously successful in increasing its share of the budgetary pie, it did have substantial political resources when it came to insulating medical education, hospital administration, and research policy from Mao's demands. The Wei-sheng-pu's two most important political resources were its capacity to narrow the range of options open to Mao (by limiting the information he received) and the symmetry of policy preferences between Ministry leaders and high-ranking central figures.

Regarding the first point, by early 1958 Mao had been disabused of any illusions he may have had regarding his ability to determine the content of bureaucratically generated policy.

> . . . the Politburo has become a voting machine, like Dulles' United Nations. You give it a perfect document and it has to be passed. Like the opera, you have to go on stage and perform since the show has been announced. The document itself does not go into textual research and essence, and it also has foreign words. I do have a method, and that is passive resistance. I will not read it.[55]

While we know very little about the strategems employed, especially during this period, it is clear that even the Chairman was in awe of the capacity of bureaucrats to foreclose his options.

Equally important was the fact that the Party Center was becoming increasingly fragmented along functional lines.[56] Those individuals with the greatest responsibility for the bureaucracy (e.g., Lu Ting-i, Teng Hsiao-p'ing, and Liu Shao-ch'i) were less willing to see it disrupted than those who had more limited responsibilities in that regard.[57] In order to make their influence effective, men like Lu Ting-i (director of the Party's Central Propaganda Department) had to establish workable, and to some extent reciprocal, relationships with ministerial leaders. We know, for instance, that Vice-Minister Ch'ien Hsin-chung was a close friend, as well as a colleague, of Lu Ting-i. Lu's continued support for high-level medical education and his opposition to a wholesale departure from previous patterns of training are understandable in terms of his bureaucratic responsibilities, his friendship

ties, and the kind of information he was probably
getting. The Wei-sheng-pu, then, could count upon
the support of some important central leaders and
its own capacity to narrow the options. While we
would like to know a great deal more about the
issues, trades, and personalities involved, what
little we do know resonates well with our knowledge
of more easily researched bureaucracies.

The Ministry leadership had to consider not
only its resources but also the resistances it faced.
The major resistance confronting it was the lethargy
which characterized the specialized bureaus in Peking
(and the duplicate structures in the provinces and
counties). For instance, attempts to reduce drug
standards would be (and were) opposed by the Bureau
of Drugs (Yao-cheng-chü).[58] Similarly, the Bureau
of Medical Education and the Ministry of Higher
Education preferred to train advanced clinicians
and researchers while local public health offices
preferred a heavier emphasis upon public health
personnel.[59] In short, while we know relatively
little about interorganizational dynamics, nothing
we do know is at variance with the operation of
other complex organizations. Within the Wei-sheng-
pu, each bureau had a defined area of specialization
and resisted policies that made the achievement of
its mission more difficult.

The perspective of prestigious physicians and
administrators also had a constraining impact. The
Chinese Academy of Medical Sciences (Chung-kuo I-
hsüeh K'o-hsüeh-yüan), a subsidiary organ of the
Ministry, expressed the view that medical education
(even before the Leap) had expanded too rapidly.
Academy members argued that this had precipitated a
decline in educational quality and facilities had
deteriorated.[60] In the Hundred Flowers period, some
doctors had called for lengthening middle-level
medical education.[61] Similarly, according to both
lab workers and doctors, pharmaceutical training,
supplies, and labs were all inadequate.[62] The quality of clinical and technical workers was said to
be particularly low, citing the example of one
druggist who mixed a toxic drug and confused "grains"
with "grams."[63]

From the perspective of the Ministry leadership,
presiding over the Wei-sheng-pu was a complex undertaking indeed. It was difficult to find a policy
alternative that would minimize intraorganizational
conflict, meet the minimal needs of doctors, and
not exceed the available resources. In general, the
most frequently pursued course was altering policy

as little as possible. Because past policy had
minimized conflict, it was most likely to do so in
the future. Change of Ministry policy tended to be
evolutionary, not revolutionary.

SUMMARY

By the end of 1958, three major health policy-
making arenas were evident. Each arena had different participants who perceived their roles, problems, and resources differently. The Central Committee (at Mao's insistence) established the Nine
Man Sub-committee on Schistosomiasis and charged
it with formulating a program for dealing with parasitic diseases. The Chairman's concern with parasitic diseases was tied to his deepening fear that
increasing rural-urban inequalities were slowing
the rate of growth and producing political instabilities. The Sub-committee, itself, was staffed
by prominent Party political personalities, all of
whom had no medical expertise. They came from areas
in which schistosomiasis was most prevalent. Party
Committees at the provincial and county levels were
responsible for implementing Sub-committee policies;
these were organs that were dominated by middle-
level cadres who attacked professionals with increasing frequency, as we shall see in the next
chapter. By late 1958, the Sub-committee had assumed
responsibility for all antiparasite programs in
China.

Health policy, as it related to the communes,
was initially formulated in the context of the
Central Committee. Mao believed that the bumper
harvests of 1958 presaged a great increase in the
resources available to rural areas; this was to
make local funding of health care possible. Every
commune (all 24,000 of them) was to have a clinic,
with administrative and policy control vested in its
Commune Party Committee. In this political arena,
middle-level upwardly mobile cadres predominated.
Policy was subject to neither the restraining influences of professionals, the central government, nor
the "masses."

The Wei-sheng-pu constituted the last of the
major arenas. Within this structure, policy-makers
were largely medical professionals who believed
that quality education and research, professional
guidance, and administrative controls were the way
to meet major difficulties. The Ministry leadership, in turn, was linked to central personalities

like Lu Ting-i and Teng Hsiao-p'ing. Each of these
men had bureaucratic ties and interests that made
them relatively responsive to arguments such as
those advanced by the Ministry. Because it was
difficult to rationalize conflicting intraorganizational demands, once policy had been agreed upon, it
tended to be resistant to change. Even as dogged an
in-fighter as Mao recognized the difficulty in making
the bureaucracy (and especially the Ministry of
Public Health) highly responsive to external pressures.

In the next chapter we shall examine the policies that emerged from these three settings, explaining the diversity of Leap policies in terms of
the particular characteristics of each arena.

NOTES

1. Kenneth Lieberthal, A Research Guide to Central
Party and Government Meetings in China: 1949-1975
(White Plains, New York: International Arts and
Sciences Press, 1976), pp. 99-121.

2. Michel Oksenberg, "The Chinese Policy Process and
the Public Health Issue: An Arena Approach,"
Studies in Comparative Communism 7, no. 4 (1974):
375-408; also, David M. Lampton, "Policy Arenas and
the Study of Chinese Politics," Studies in Comparative Communism 7, no. 4 (1974):409-413.

3. David M. Lampton, "Health Policy During the
Great Leap Forward," China Quarterly (hereafter CQ),
no. 60 (1974), pp. 669-698.

4. Audrey Donnithorne, China's Economic System (New
York: Praeger, 1967), p. 130.

5. "Ch'üan-kuo Fang-chih Hsüeh-chi-hsiung-ping
Hui-i Tsai Shang-hai Chu-hsing" [National antischis-
tosomiasis meeting convened in Shanghai], Kuang-ming
Jih-pao [Bright daily], April 7, 1956.

6. Donald W. Klein and Anne B. Clark, Dictionary
of Chinese Communism (Cambridge: Harvard University
Press, 1971), pp. 440-441.

7. "Fang-chih Hsüeh-chi-hsiung-ping Chan-hsien-
shang Te Hsin Sheng-li" [A new victory in the battle
to prevent schistosomiasis], Jen-min Jih-pao
[People's daily], May 16, 1958.

8. Who's Who in Communist China (Hong Kong: Union Research Institute, 1970), p. 711.

9. David M. Lampton, Interview File 21.

10. David M. Lampton, Interview File 21 C.

11. Michel Oksenberg, unpublished chronology.

12. Kuang-ming Jih-pao [Bright daily], April 7, 1956; see also, Kuang-ming Jih-pao [Bright daily], July 6, 1958.

13. Mao Tse-tung, Miscellany of Mao Tse-tung Thought (1949-1968), Joint Publications Research Service, no. 61269-1 (February 20, 1974), pp. 172-173.

14. "Thorough Prevention and Cure of Schistosomiasis," Jen-min Jih-pao [People's daily], January 22, 1957, in Survey of the China Mainland Press (hereafter SMCP), no. 1473, p. 15.

15. For the resolution of the August 1958 Pei-tai-ho Conference see, Jen-min Shou-ts'e [People's handbook] (Peking: Ta-kung-she, 1959), pp. 32-34. At the Sixth Plenum of the Eighth Central Committee in December 1958, Mao said that communes were not "discovered" until August. "The appearance of the people's communes was not foreseen at the Ch'engtu Conference in April [sic. March] and the Party Congress in May. Actually it had already appeared in Honan in April, but remained unknown through May, June, and July until its discovery in August. . . ." Mao Tse-tung, "Tsai Pa-chü Liu Chung Ch'üan-hui-i-shang Te Chiang-hua" [Speech at the Sixth Plenum], Mao Tse-tung, Mao Tse-tung Ssu-hsiang Wan-sui [Long live the thought of Mao Tse-tung] (Peking: 1969), p. 259.

16. Donnithorne, pp. 66-67.

17. Li Teh-hua and Yang Min-ting, "The Planning of Ch'ingpu Hsien and Hung Ch'i People's Commune," Current Background (hereafter CB), no. 544, p. 8.

18. Ezra Vogel, Interview No. 42, p. 2.

19. David M. Lampton, Interview File 21 C.

20. Mao Tse-tung, "Tsai Nan-ning Hui-i-shang Te Chiang-hua" [Speech at the Nanning Conference], Mao

<u>Tse-tung Ssu-hsiang Wan-sui</u>, p. 153.

21. Mao Tse-tung, "Lun Shih Ta Kuan-hsi" [On the ten great relationships], <u>Mao Tse-tung Ssu-hsiang Wan-sui</u>, pp. 40-59.

22. Mao Tse-tung, "On the Correct Handling of Contradictions Among the People," <u>Selected Readings from the Works of Mao Tse-tung</u> (Peking: Foreign Languages Press, 1971), p. 476.

23. <u>Shansi Jih-pao</u> [Shansi daily], March 20, 1957. This article noted that peasants resented paying for medical care at cooperative clinics and having to pay extra for night calls.

24. <u>New China News Agency</u> (hereafter <u>NCNA</u>), May 14, 1957. Cited in, Roderick MacFarquhar, <u>The Hundred Flowers</u> (London: Stevens and Sons, Ltd., 1960), p. 233.

25. Sun Kuang, "Urban Population Must be Controlled," <u>Jen-min Jih-pao</u> [People's daily], November 27, 1957, in <u>SCMP</u>, no. 1668, pp. 5 and 7.

26. Mao Tse-tung, "Tsai Pa Ta Erh-ts'e Hui-i-shang Te Chiang-hua: Ti Erh-ts'e Chiang-hua" [Speech at the Second Session of the Eighth Central Committee: the second speech], <u>Mao Tse-tung Ssu-hsiang Wan-sui</u>, p. 201.

27. Mao Tse-tung, "Preface to Socialist Upsurge in China's Countryside," <u>Hsin Jen Wei</u> [New people's health] (Peking: People's Health Press, 1967), pp. 9-10.

28. David M. Lampton, <u>Health, Conflict, and the Chinese Political System</u>, Papers in Chinese Studies, no. 18 (Ann Arbor: Center for Chinese Studies, University of Michigan, 1974), Chapter 2.

29. <u>NCNA</u>, May 14, 1957. Cited in MacFarquhar, p. 233.

30. <u>Jen-min Jih-pao</u> [People's daily], October 6, 1956. Cited in MacFarquhar, p. 127.

31. <u>Chien-k'ang Pao</u> [Health bulletin], January 18, 1957.

32. <u>Chien-k'ang Pao</u> [Health bulletin], May 7, 1957.

33. Sun Kuang, p. 7.

34. Ezra Vogel, Canton Under Communism (Cambridge: Harvard University Press, 1969), p. 259.

35. Ezra Vogel, Interview No. 19, p. 2.

36. Hsi Yeh-tun, "Ch'üan-kuo I-yüan Kung-tso Hui-i-shang Te Chung-ta I-i" [The great significance of the National Hospital Work Conference], I-hsüeh Shih Yü Pao-chien Tsu-chih [Medical history and health organization], no. 1 (1958), p. 23. This document called upon hospitals to eliminate "unnecessary" laboratory tests and noted that patient living standards were "divorced from the standard of living of the people."

37. Ho Piao, "Tsai Ch'üan-kuo I-yüan Kung-tso Hui-i-shang Te Pao-kao" [Report to the National Hospital Work Conference], Hsin-hua Pan-yüeh-k'an [New China semi-monthly], no. 128 (March 1958), pp. 143-148.

38. Sheng-yang Jih-pao [Shengyang daily], January 9, 1957.

39. Chien-k'ang Pao [Health bulletin], May 7, 1957.

40. Li Teh-hua and Yang Min-ting.

41. Chu-yuan Cheng, "Health Manpower: Growth and Distribution," Public Health in the People's Republic of China, ed. Myron E. Wegman, Tsung-yi Lin, and Elizabeth Purcell (New York: Macy Foundation, 1973), p. 145.

42. Chien-k'ang Pao [Health bulletin], January 18, 1957, p. 2.

43. Mao Tse-tung, "Tsai Ch'eng-tu Hui-i-shang Te Chiang-hua" [Speech at the Ch'engtu Conference], Mao Tse-tung Ssu-hsiang Wan-sui, p. 161.

44. Mao Tse-tung, Miscellany, p. 89.

45. Wen-hui Pao, September 29, 1958.

46. Mao Tse-tung, "Tsai Ch'eng-tu Hui-i-shang Te Chiang-hua" [Speech at the Ch'engtu Conference], Mao Tse-tung Ssu-hsiang Wan-sui, p. 161.

47. Thomas P. Bernstein, "Leadership and Mass Mobilization in the Soviet and Chinese

Collectivization Campaigns of 1929-30 and 1955-56:
A Comparison," CQ, no. 31 (1967), p. 2.

48. Mao Tse-tung, Miscellany, p. 88.

49. Wen-hui Pao, March 10, 1959.

50. "Yao-ts'ai Sheng-ch'an Chien" [Drug production
declines], Hsiang-kang Shih-pao [Hong Kong times],
November 10, 1958.

51. Hsi Yeh-tun, p. 23.

52. This is based upon an extrapolation from an
overall decline in the culture, education, and health
portion of the budget of about 6 percent. Up until
1956, the health component of this portion of the
budget maintained a constant share. I presume
declines were proportionally shared by the health,
education, and culture organizations. See Nai-ruenn
Chen, p. 446.

53. Michel Oksenberg, Interviews Nos. 1 and 2; see
also, Ezra Vogel, Canton Under Communism, p. 225.

54. Nicholas R. Lardy, "Centralization and Decentralization in China's Fiscal Management," CQ, no.
61 (1975), p. 37.

55. Mao Tse-tung, "Tsai Nan-ning Hui-i-shang Te
Chiang-hua" [Speech at the Nanning Conference], Mao
Tse-tung Ssu-hsiang Wan-sui, p. 149.

56. A. Doak Barnett, Cadres, Bureaucracy, and
Political Power in Communist China (New York:
Columbia University Press, 1967), pp. 4-10.

57. "Mayflies Lightly Plot to Topple Giant Tree,"
Ch'üan-wu-ti [Invincible], June 26, 1967, in Survey
of the China Mainland Press-Supplement, no. 209,
pp. 14-23.

58. Chien-k'ang Pao [Health bulletin], May 7, 1957,
p. 1.

59. Chien-k'ang Pao [Health bulletin], May 7, 1957,
p. 1.

60. Chien-k'ang Pao [Health bulletin], May 17, 1957;
see also, Ezra Vogel, Interview No. 21, p. 1.

61. "Kuan-yü I-shih Hsüeh-hsiao Te Chi-ko Wen-t'i"
[A few problems concerning medical school], Chien-
k'ang Pao [Health bulletin], April 5, 1957.

62. Chien-k'ang Pao [Health bulletin], April 5, 1957,
p. 2; see also, Chien-k'ang Pao [Health bulletin],
January 18, 1957.

63. "We Must Change the Tendency to Lightly Regard
Hospital Pharmaceutical Work," Chien-k'ang Pao
[Health bulletin], April 2, 1957.

97

Chapter 5
THE CONSEQUENCES OF
EXCESSIVE DIVISION OF AUTHORITY:
THE POLICIES AND PROBLEMS
OF THE LEAP

INTRODUCTION

By the end of 1958, there were three relatively independent forums in which health policy was being made. In this chapter, we shall briefly outline the decisions and the personalities that sustained this "divided system" and then analyze the policy consequences of this arrangement. The argument to follow is simply this: Persons in the Central Committee and the Politburo having daily responsibility for the bureaucracy tried to insulate the Ministry, as much as possible, from the turmoil of the other policy-making arenas. Chou En-lai's role at the Third Plenum (September-October 1957) was particularly important. By January 1958 (the Nanning Conference), Mao had acknowledged that the ministries would continue to act largely as they had in the past; his concerns, and those of his colleagues in the Central Committee, would be fixed upon the transformation of the rural sector.

The major difficulty with this kind of division of authority was that policy areas were interlocking and that mass campaign activities, for instance, had an impact on communes, county hospitals, and drug producers. Similarly, the creation of commune clinics on a vast scale had important implications for the educational apparatus, as well as drug and equipment manufacturers. In short, bureaucratic action in one issue area could not be insulated from action in the other two policy-making arenas. The result was a lack of program coordination and the ultimate collapse of the Leap itself. This chapter will develop this case by looking at seven specific issue areas.

Because the Leap collapsed due to the inability of policy-makers and implementors to achieve coordination, we must specify how this division of labor occurred. Unfortunately, many of the most interesting questions must remain unanswered until more detailed documentation becomes available.

The times at which decisive moves toward a division of labor occurred were the Third Plenum of the Eighth Central Committee (September-October 1957)[1] and the Nanning Conference of January 1958.[2] At the Third Plenum, Premier Chou En-lai made a major speech in which he dealt with questions of health care. While no complete transcript of this speech has been released, two summaries are available.[3] The traditional view of the Third Plenum has been that it laid the foundation for the efforts of the Leap. Vogel notes,

> The Third Plenum . . . was a crucial turning point. It ended almost two years of wavering and debate over basic policy and initiated a concerted and ultimately utopian effort to cut short the process of modernization by moral suasion, sacrifice, and physical labor.[4]

Recently available documentation, however, makes it clear that consensus was not achieved at the Third Plenum. There was stiff opposition to "bold advances." As Mao said at the subsequent Nanning Conference,

> At the Third Plenary Session of the Central Committee I said that three things were abolished last year [greater, faster, better, and more economical results, the forty articles, and the promotion committees] and there was no opposition. . . . I then had the courage to talk to the Ministers again. There has been a setback in these three years. The rightists launched full-scale opposition against "bold advances" . . .[5]

Chou's Third Plenum speech has to be seen in this context. He was trying to insulate the ministries (as much as possible) while not appearing obstructionist. Premier Chou laid down five policy guidelines for health care: (1) Health care should serve everyone, city and countryside alike. (This formulation was caustically rejected in the

99

Cultural Revolution.) (2) Preventive health work should be strengthened, thereby cutting demand for hospitalization. (3) The excessive purchase of equipment should be halted but, the ". . . necessary cures and the use of necessary drugs cannot be reduced, [we] must guarantee medical quality."[6] (4) Health facilities should stay open longer and be more convenient for the peasants. (5) Finally, Chou cautioned against moving toward consolidated management units (through "united management") too rapidly.

Each of these points will be analyzed in the discussions of particular policies, but, a few general remarks are in order. First, Chou avoided thorny issues of allocation by assuring that city and countryside would receive equal ("ch'eng hsiang chien ku") treatment.[7] Secondly, the statement appears to have been designed to assure the Ministry leadership and physicians that their legitimate requests for drugs and equipment would be honored, though they were expected to resist the temptation to make non-essential purchases. Thirdly, the premier tried to prevent the health system from changing its administrative structure too rapidly; he was a restraining influence. The points relating to making medical facilities more convenient and promoting prevention were nothing more than restatements of operative Ministry policy. Concisely, Chou was calling for added administrative efficiency, not fundamental transformation of the Wei-sheng-pu.

As mentioned in the previous chapter, two months later at the Nanning Conference, Chairman Mao acknowledged that a division of policy-making authority existed.[8] His eyes (and those of the Central Committee) were focused on the rural areas. The State Council was to continue administering the ministries as it had previously.

While there is much that we do not know, one hypothesis that resonates with the available data is that a compromise had been agreed to in which the technical organizations in the State Council would permit radicalization of policy in the rural sector in exchange for relative stability in their domains. Chou's Third Plenum speech appears to be a political document in the truest sense of the word. He was trying to be all things to all men. He reassured the bureaucrats and professionals that they would be called upon to make only minimal changes. For those demanding more substantial alterations, he portrayed his requests as fundamental. In any case, by 1958 there were three policy-making arenas, a

fact that was pregnant with consequences for the
next several years.

GREAT LEAP ACTION POLICIES

Medical education's fundamental policy statement was enunciated by Premier Chou En-lai at the
Third Plenum, and was formally adopted by Vice-
Minister of Public Health Ho Piao in his March 1958
speech to the National Hospital Work Conference.
Neither of these statements was very specific, but
both called for an increased emphasis on middle-
level medical schools. At the time these speeches
were delivered, between 15,000 and 20,000 middle-
level doctors were being produced each year.[9] By
1960, the number of students enrolled in such
schools was announced to have increased to about
150,000, indicating a yearly graduation rate of
50,000.[10] Most (if not all) of these schools were
under county or provincial control. One would like
to know how many secondary medical schools were
built during the Leap, but the available figures
are incomplete and contradictory. The only conclusion at which one can safely arrive is that enrollments in middle medical schools increased by
approximately 100 percent. Those schools which were
new often were small, poorly equipped and staffed,
and highly dependent upon local financing. As local
financing went, so went these institutions.
Higher medical education (until 1959) was not
the subject of any directive which is presently
available. Curriculum length remained the same as
it had in previous years, despite the fact that Mao
had apparently called for a reduction in the length
of training sometime in 1958.[11] In the absence of
precise documentation for both Mao's directive and
the Wei-sheng-pu's response, we cannot be specific
except to note that the Ministry did not alter
higher-level medical schools in any fundamental way.
The major burden that fell upon these medical
schools was having to admit more students; enrollments may have increased by 25-30 percent, with an
undetermined percentage of the increase coming from
students of working-class background.

From 1958-1959, due to shortage in building
materials and rooms, there has not been a
general expansion of positions in the universities and this is particularly complicated by
the fact that a number of students from the

101

working class who are now forced to be admitted particularly since 1958-1959 by demand of the country, make it difficult for the usual student to get in.[12]

As early as December 1958, the Leap's difficulties became apparent and the Chairman admitted that he had been overenthusiastic at the Pei-tai-ho Conference and that the education question would have to be discussed at "the February Meeting"[13] in Ch'engchow. Trends toward moderation were equally visible at the Sixth Plenum of November-December 1958.[14] Just prior to the Sixth Plenum, Mao noted that a role for technicians had to be recognized because "industry is different from agriculture. In industry, many factors affect one another through their mutual relationships. . . . There can be no missing link."[15] In short, by early 1959, while there was yet a hesitance to back off from radical agrarian policies, there was a recognition that the insulation of the technical spheres had to be substantial. Following the Second Ch'engchow Conference (February 1959), Chou En-lai made a major speech in which he directed medical educators to improve the level of training in "key schools."

> Full-time regular schools at all levels should make it their constant and fundamental task to raise the quality of teaching and studying; in the first place, we must devote relatively more energy to perfecting a number of "key" schools so as to train specialized personnel of higher quality for the state and bring about a rapid rise in our country's scientific and cultural level.[16]

By early 1959, in response to this encouragement, the Ministry of Health and the Ministry of Higher Education boosted curriculum length in major medical schools, like Peking Medical College and Shanghai First Medical College, to six years, with the prestigious China Medical College lengthening it to eight years. In addition, the China Union Medical College was placed under the direct control of the Chinese Academy of Medical Sciences, an organization dominated by professionals. The combined effect of professional displeasure, the technical problems of the Leap itself, and the insulation of the Ministry policy-making apparatus meant that higher-level medical education had been able to resist the worst excesses of the Leap in 1958;

once it faltered in early 1959, the Wei-sheng-pu
was able to push medical standards to higher levels
than ever before. In sum, while mobilizational
agrarian, mass campaign, and urban commune policies
were still being pursued, medical education was
moving in the opposite direction.

Medical doctors and educators, however, could
not remain entirely insulated from the Leap. Provincial Party Committees and Provincial People's
Committees assigned an unknown number of regular
and middle-level doctors to go to county medical
facilities to train rural "health workers."

> 225 doctors or feldshers and others were chosen
> for this purpose by the Provincial Party Com-
> mittee and the Provincial People's Committee.
> After two months' training, they were sent . . .
> to the different endemic counties to train
> others. . . .[17]

In Shanghai, this program began in 1958; the health
workers which were trained were assigned to production brigades and became "barefoot doctors" (ch'ih-
chiao i-sheng).[18]

The question of prime interest is, what were
the political dynamics which led to this array of
educational policies? Within the Ministry, financial resources were limited and the prestige schools
were under its direct control. As we noted in the
first chapter, the Ministry had always had the
incentive to give as many responsibilities as possible to lower levels while minimizing its allocations
to them. With the financial constraints of 1958,
the Ministry had even more need to insulate the
major medical schools from disruption. In financial
and bureaucratic terms, the expansion of activities
at the county and provincial levels is understandable, just as is the relative continuity in higher-
level medical education.

There are additional political factors that
played a role in facilitating the insulation of
higher-level medical education. On the question of
"key" institutions, there appears to have been a
division of opinion (in 1958) among the top leadership. That year, the Chairman issued a directive
saying, "Education must serve proletarian politics
and education must be combined with productive
labor." At about the same time, Mao said, "The
period of schooling should be shortened. . . ."[19]
In contrast, Lu Ting-i (director of propaganda and
vice-premier of the State Council) and Liu Shao-ch'i

are accused of having argued that some educational institutions should have longer curricula.[20]   While we know very little about this debate, Chou En-lai's speech to the Third Plenum and his address to the First Session of the Second National People's Congress (March 1959), seem to have reflected the compromises which had been worked out.   While neither Liu nor Lu were able to implement their desires for longer education in the face of Mao's opposition, they were able to prevent Mao from implementing his.   Once the Chairman began to waver on his policies at the Sixth Plenum, these individuals were able to implement policies they and medical professionals in the Wei-sheng-pu had favored all along.   Just where Mao stood at this juncture is still unclear.   Two conclusions emerge from even these limited data: First, many more people in the Chinese political system can effectively veto a policy than implement one.   Secondly, there was a clear trend toward cooptation and bureaucratic "representation."   It would appear to be no accident that Lu Ting-i, Liu Shao-ch'i, and Chou En-lai, the three individuals most intimately concerned with the bureaucracy and professionals, were the most forceful advocates of higher medical education standards.

Great Leap policy vis à vis medical research followed the broad contours of educational policy, though the degree of insulation may have been greater.   The indications of a relatively "pro-research" bias are numerous.   The number of medical conferences held in China reached an all time high in 1959 (see Appendix D); it was the anti-rightist campaign of 1957-1958 that most reduced the number of conferences being held.   Similarly, the president of the Chinese Medical Association noted that an increasing number of journals was being published. Fourteen medical journals were in circulation at that time and the number of "pure" (or "exotic") research articles carried in the Chinese Medical Journal was as high as ever.   Appendix B shows that during the 1955-April 1957 period, 74 percent of each issue of the average Chinese Medical Journal was devoted to articles dealing with "exotic" medical subjects.   With the "wilting" of the Hundred Flowers Campaign in May and June 1957, the number of pure research articles declined markedly, only to rise to almost the old levels throughout the remainder of the year.   During 1958, the space devoted to sophisticated medical research remained at these levels, except when major central meetings

were in progress (see Appendix B).[21] While the
simultaneous occurrence of these meetings and
declines in high-level research articles might be
coincidental, a logical inference is that medical
research continued "normally" and that officials of
the Chinese Medical Association and the Wei-sheng-pu
merely increased or decreased the rate of publication depending on the political weather. If this
occurred, it would be consistent with the hypothesis
that what we are seeing is an insulated research
apparatus trying to protect itself.

Not only did research remain relatively insulated, it also acquired additional areas of responsibility. This was done at the expense of the
Academy of Traditional Medicine (Chung-i Yen-chiu-
yüan). In January 1957, an article appeared in
Chien-k'ang Pao (Health bulletin) calling for the
transferral of responsibility for pharmaceutical
and clinical research from the Academy of Traditional Medicine to the Chinese Academy of Medical Sciences, because the past performance of traditional
researchers allegedly had been low.[22] This proposal
was tabled during the subsequent anti-rightist campaign but was adopted as Ministry policy in March
1959.[23] In short, during a movement in which traditional medicine was being promoted on one level (the
mass campaign level), it was being restricted on
another (the research level).

There is one other indirect indication that
research maintained continuity with the past; brain
and heart surgery, along with the treatment of
massive burns and traumatic amputations, made substantial strides.[24] Interviews indicate that while
the rhetoric of mass participation in research was
evident, in fact, each major research team had a
core group of professionals who conducted business
as near to usual as possible. As Minister of Health
Li Teh-ch'uan noted in April 1959,

> As a result, certain previously weak links in
> medical science have been strengthened. For
> instance, heart surgery and brain surgery have
> developed considerably.[25]

While there are no data indicating the magnitude of allocations for medical research, one would
guess that they probably stayed near old levels.
Only the economic fiasco of 1960 would really hurt
research. As noted previously, it was possible for
research funds to increase while the Ministry's budget declined because of "independent" funding

through the Academy of Sciences. In short, there
may have been financial reasons for the insulation
of medical research.

One should note that medical researchers and
professionals had a pervasive influence on science
policy-making, even during the Leap. They were
heavily represented in the Academy of Sciences, the
Academy of Medical Sciences, and the Ministry's
Scientific Committee on Medical Sciences. One
knowledgeable interviewee reported that even a newly
created organ to oversee research policy, the State
Scientific and Technological Commission (Kuo-wu-yüan
K'o-hsüeh Chi-shu Wei-yüan-hui), "was promoting
science."[26] Besides direct professional impact,
Chou En-lai argued for maintaining high standards
in research, saying,

> Attention must also be given to developing the
> most advanced branches of science and tech-
> nology; as regards those branches in which we
> lack conditions for development, we must make
> all the necessary preparations now. Basic
> theoretic research exerts a far-reaching influ-
> ence on scientific and technological progress,
> and we must pay sufficient attention to this
> field as well.[27]

In sum, the insulation of medical research
reflected the initial division of labor that had
been agreed to in 1957-1958, the relatively stronger
institutional position of researchers in State Council organs, the support of powerful central figures,
and the probable differences between Wei-sheng-pu
and medical research financing. As in education,
the radical rhetoric of the mass campaigns and communes is not always a good indicator of the policy
emerging from the bureaucracy. The mass media tend
to overemphasize discontinuity, making it easy to
overlook the many continuities that are always
present.

Policy regarding the health delivery system was
one issue area in which substantial change occurred,
though there were continuities which are significant
as well. In the cities, the Wei-sheng-pu apparatus
continued to administer the hospitals while Commune
Party Committees were responsible for such tasks in
the newly established rural hospitals and clinics.

In urban areas (down to, and including, the
county), the Ministry continued to promote the "sectional medical service." Each urban hospital was
responsible for serving all the people in its

geographic area and each medical facility had a special responsibility for workers in factories with which it had contracts. This is true in 1977 as well. Workers could not go to the hospital without first obtaining the permission of the responsible factory medical officer. One primary function of this system was to reduce the number of cases referred to hospitals.

> . . . rational adjustments of medical service contracts and proper organization of the masses of the people have eased the congestion at the larger hospitals. . . .[28]

Despite this attempt to reduce the burdens on urban hospitals, several forces kept straining hospital facilities. While we have no statistical data, it is clear from interviews and later reports that the combined effect of the communes and the mass campaigns was to increase the patient burdens of urban hospitals.[29] With the dearth of money and the shortage of building materials, local hospitals were unable to expand their facilities (even if there had been time). As a consequence, all hospitals could do was to increase patient censuses. This produced crowding and the quality of service deteriorated. Because elite sectors of the society (e.g., Party and government cadres) had been major users of the medical system, this represented a net decline in the quality of care they received. Such individuals were among the most anxious to see pre-Leap standards restored.

Changes in the rural delivery system were much more substantial. Each of China's approximately 24,000 communes was to have a medical clinic. By mid-1959, Minister of Health Li Teh-ch'uan noted that about half the nation's communes had functioning medical facilities;[30] by 1960 it was alleged the remaining units had some type of clinic.[31] Many, if not most, rural clinics were the old united clinics for which the commune now assumed financial responsibility. While the provinces and counties did try to allocate medical personnel to these units, it took time to train them. Consequently, in the short-run, commune clinics were still largely staffed by traditional practitioners. Therefore, while the communes did change the organizational and financial context of rural medical delivery, they did not immediately change the quality of rural service. This explains why such clinics were so easily abandoned when the financial squeeze hit in the early 1960s.

107

An important determinant of the availability of health care was the availability and cost of pharmaceuticals. Without an adequate drug supply, the effectiveness of any health delivery system is reduced. In 1958, there was a 34 percent reduction in the price of drugs.[32] This was a move that had heretofore been resisted by the Chemical and Commercial Ministries because they feared that demand for drugs would increase too rapidly. Once prices were reduced, demand skyrocketed. As the Chinese Medical Journal delicately put it,

> The setting up of clinics and health stations following the establishment of people's communes in the vast countryside, and the nationwide mass movements to wipe out the four pests, improve sanitary conditions, and eliminate the principal diseases, coupled with the rise in the people's living standard, created a formidable proposition for our pharmaceutical industry.[33]

These price reductions precipitated declines in the quality and standardization of drugs to the point that doctors hesitated to prescribe them.[34] In 1960, the Pharmaceutical Association felt compelled to note that the government was concerned about drug quality as well as availability.[35]

Once again, we have seen policy diversity within what superficially appears to have been a homogeneous movement. Changes within the urban hospital system were administrative and not particularly fundamental. This was the case because of the financial limitations and the inability to expand service without lowering quality. The kind of manpower needed to staff a complex hospital system could not be created over night. The increased burdens being placed on medical facilities just aggravated the problem which had always faced the Wei-sheng-pu; how could waste and overutilization be limited? Of course, any attempt to deny some persons access (or reduce the quality of service rendered) was bound to alienate the affected portion of the population. Herein lies the basis for hostility against the health system.

In rural areas, changes in the delivery system were much more substantial. At no time in Chinese history had the government promoted a program designed to bring "free" health care to the peasantry. As we shall see shortly, the new financial system, combined with anticipated increases in agricultural production, was supposed to make this possible. The commune clinics, however, did not make the services of western-style doctors immediately available. Traditional practitioners still predominated in these facilities. Because the capabilities of rural personnel and facilities were limited, the commune clinics often functioned as conduits, referring more patients to urban hospitals than these institutions could handle. To commune cadres, however, these were the problems of the hospital system. Only changes in local leadership, financial relationships, and referral regulations could change this.

Financial policy. As noted earlier, the counties and provinces had been the "victims" of past policies; they had always been given more tasks to perform than revenue with which to carry them out. In order to obtain the necessary funds, local units had been forced to levy "self-help" taxes. As a former Ministry of Finance employee noted, this method of local financing alienated the peasants.

> This method of levying taxes was not much different from the KMT method and the peasants were being alienated as a result. The irregularity of the tax system, with lack of thorough reporting, etc., easily led to corrupt practices. Thus, the 1958 regulations forbid the tzu-ch'ou [self-help] system, and gave hsien and hsiang a set income and set scope for taxation.[36]

As noted earlier, however, regularizing local revenues was not necessarily the same as increasing their total. The research already cited indicates that, in fact, local units acquired few additional resources; they had vastly more burdens thrust upon them. This is one of the major reasons for the severe insolvency of many county facilities during this period.[37] Urban population increased rapidly and more peasants were coming to county health facilities. The result was that hospital costs went up and, as agricultural production faltered in 1959 and 1960, an increasing number of bills remained unpaid. As the agricultural crisis deepened in 1960 and 1961, these difficulties became more severe.

> Communes are theoretically supposed to pay for the workers [peasants] to go to the county hospital but there has been a lot of difficulty in getting more money out of the communes

109

and county hospitals have lost a lot of money by treating commune patients.[38]

The innovative aspect of medical care financing occurred in the communes. While there were many variants of financial plans, some involving patient contributions, two types of plans were particularly common. In financial plan Type I, production brigades established a welfare fund made up of revenues from brigade enterprises and agricultural production. Additionally, the commune remitted a set sum of money to the brigade (pao-kan i-liao).[39] The brigade fund was responsible for covering the expenses of its people at commune and above health facilities. Under financial plan Type II, the commune, itself, set aside funds for health care and paid for all commune members.[40]

Three difficulties arose in the course of trying to provide "free," or highly subsidized, medical care to all peasants: (1) Relatively well-to-do brigades and teams often wanted to have their own system and did not wish to subsidize less prosperous units. (2) Relatively well-to-do individuals frequently were reticent to support a welfare fund which was basically redistributive. (3) It was difficult to control costs because individuals bore no economic burden for overutilization. All these factors tended to create disincentive effects in the production sphere and produce program insolvency. Regarding the first two problems, one article noted,

> There was in the May 1 Production Team a commune member who thought in the past that since he was physically strong and full of energy and his family was comparatively well-off economically, the enforcement of cooperative medical service would benefit other people at his own expenses.[41]

Donnithorne notes, ". . . the disincentive effects of such a tendency [toward commune welfare] on the more prosperous brigades provoked a reaction and warnings were issued against egalitarianism."[42]

Inability to control costs was the major problem with "free" commune medical care, as we shall see in the next two chapters. The immediate response, however, was to transfer some of the financial burden back onto users by levying mandatory contributions and use fees. As Red Flag summed up ten years later, placing charges on the individual ". . . fits in with the present rural economic

110

basis . . . and with our country's rural economic
level."[43]

Great Leap financial policy in the communes
reflected many pressures, constraints, and perceived
opportunities. Peasants wanted health care and the
Party believed that provision of such services would
forestall further alienation. At the same time,
central and local monetary resources were limited.
In 1958, anticipated increases in agricultural production looked like the way to cut this Gordian
knot. A portion of the new wealth could be siphoned
off to pay for welfare services through the device
of brigade and commune welfare funds.

Once agricultural increases failed to material-
ize, however, the financial plans which were dependent upon such increases became unworkable. Agricultural declines forced local cadres to push costs
off onto either consumers and/or higher levels.
Communes and their constituent production brigades
referred patients to county facilities and then
balked at paying for them.[44] The Leap had consequences for hospitals that were the opposite of
those intended.

The fact that demands for medical services were
escalating rapidly was apparent as early as April
1959. Li Hsien-nien announced a planned increase
of 32 percent in health, education, and culture
expenditures for 1959. Health, education, and culture planned expenditures rose from 4,350 million ¥
in 1958 to 5,730 million ¥ in 1959.[45] By the end
of 1959, even this amount had been exceeded by 130
million ¥.[46] These expenditures had to be weighed
against the spectre of precipitously declining
revenues and competing needs, especially those of
defense, agriculture, and industry. In 1959, the
percentage of the budget allocated to health, education, and culture reached an historic high while
defense expenditures reached their nadir. What
impact this had on General P'eng Teh-huai's attack
on the Leap as "petty bourgeois fanaticism" is
unknown, but, the sequence of events is suggestive.
Roderick MacFarquhar has documented P'eng's long-
standing position that defense expenditures had to
be maintained at relatively high levels.[47]

Policy with respect to the conditions of physician employment was subject to contradictory
pressures, pressures which were least burdensome in
elite medical and research institutes. Doctors, in
their capacity as clinicians and teachers, fared
somewhat differently. The fact that physicians had
three primary roles produced role ambiguity and
conflict.

111

Clinicians witnessed the greatest change in
their working conditions as the number of patients
for whom they were responsible rapidly grew. Doctors
often had to see thirty to fifty patients per day,
which meant that neither the doctor nor the patient
was very happy. As drugs became increasingly scarce
and less reliable, patients often requested pharmaceuticals of foreign manufacture, a desire that
physicians were generally unable to satisfy. Doctors, still vulnerable to accusations of "harboring
class resentment" when the requests of "working-
class" people had to be denied, hesitated to assume
the responsibility for ending waste and "frivolous"
use. Those denied service could frequently make
their lives miserable. Within hospitals, the hierarchy of authority began to weaken; paramedics,
nurses, and other hospital personnel were encouraged
by Party zealots to engage in activities which
doctors considered far beyond their competence.[48]

Physicians sought ways to make themselves less
vulnerable to political attack and ways to reduce
"interference" in their work. During the Leap,
joining the Youth League or the Communist Party was
one way to do this. The Party was receptive to
such applications, though apparently not on the
scale that it had been in 1956.[49]

Doctors, in their role as educators, fared
somewhat better. Prestigious medical schools had
remained relatively insulated, even during 1958;
with the emphasis on "key schools" in early 1959,
they fared even better. Admissions standards were
maintained and curricula length extended. In non-
elite medical schools, however, the size of classes
increased and there appears to have been a more
pronounced bias toward "working-class" recruitment.[50]

Another force for potential "disruption" in
medical education was the November 18, 1958 Central
Committee directive that full-time Chung-i courses
for western-style doctors be established; 2,000
physicians were to be involved.[51] Neither the
Ministry nor the medical profession was enthusiastic
about such a policy and they both sought to scotch
any thought of making the study of Chung-i mandatory
for all physicians. In agreeing to the Central
Committee's call for additional emphasis on Chung-i,
Dr. Fu Lien-chang, head of the Chinese Medical
Association and a respected doctor from the Kiangsi
Soviet period, said, ". . . we should also call on
other western-style doctors to take up part-time
study, where feasible, on a voluntary basis and on
the principle of studying their own specialties.

112

But we should not require all western-style doctors
unconditionally to study traditional medicine. This
would add more difficulties to their already heavy
burden of work."[52] The policy which was finally implemented was that each doctor would study Chung-i
part-time for three months. Once again, professional and Ministry opinion influenced the final
shape of policy, though these forces certainly did
not win an unconditional victory.

Doctors, as medical researchers in the Academy
of Sciences and the Academy of Medical Sciences,
enjoyed the least encumbered existence. They had
sources of revenue which were, to some extent, im-
mune from the constraints being placed on the Wei-
sheng-pu. Also, while we can't speak with authority
about the last months of 1958, by April 1959 Premier
Chou had made advanced scientific research a major
government priority.[53] As noted above, Li Teh-ch'uan
observed that gains had been made in heart and
brain surgery and more professional conferences were
held in 1959 than ever before.

In sum, the more prestigious the institution in
which the doctor worked, and the more research oriented his position within the profession, the less
he was affected by Great Leap Forward mobilization.
The most disrupted physician was the one in a clinic
or hospital at the provincial or county level where
professional contacts were least numerous and patient loads more burdensome.

Policy vis à vis traditional medicine was the
result of a subtle interplay of leadership cleavages,
goals, resources, and social pressures. Because of
the increased demand for medical services during the
Great Leap Forward, everyone seemed to see some need
to utilize the services of traditional doctors, if
for no other reason than they staffed the bulk of
commune clinics. Additionally, Vice-Ministers Hsu
Yun-pei and Chang Kai had gained their positions in
a dispute over traditional medicine; one presumes
they would have been most committed to this issue.
Finally, even Ministry professionals had to bolster
the status of Chung-i to the point where the rural
populace would settle for treatment in commune
clinics rather than flooding urban facilities.

Policy in this area dealt with four broad issue
areas: (1) Increased study, by western-style doctors, of Chinese medical theory. (2) The integration of traditional practitioners into western-style
medical facilities. (3) The construction of traditional medical schools. (4) Increased research into
traditional curative practices and pharmaceuticals.

Professional resistance to these programs was greatest in the first area and less pronounced as one
approached the last category.

Quite predictably, having Chung-i incorporated
in western-style medical curricula met with the most
resistance from both modern practitioners and traditional physicians. This policy was hard to insti-
tutionalize because neither western nor traditional-
style doctors had a perceived stake in it. While
it is understandable why modern doctors would resist
such a policy, it may be less clear why traditional
doctors would. Traditional practitioners viewed the
dispersal of their skills as a threat to their
livelihood. One practitioner noted,

> The Ministry's present policy with respect to
> Chung-i, from the present point of view, has
> substituted the past "rightism" [of Wang Pin]
> for the "leftism" of allowing those who were
> not previously Chinese practitioners, and who
> have not studied Chinese medicine, to now
> become Chinese doctors. . . .[54]

Not only were traditional practitioners opposed
to the policy of widely teaching traditional curative techniques, but, as we have seen, so was the
western-style medical community. The Central Committee's November 18, 1958 directive had had the
potentially sharp edges removed before implementation. In short, forcing western-style doctors to
study traditional medicine had very little bureaucratic or professional constituency. As one would
predict, it was one of the least durable dimensions
of health policy.

The attempt to integrate traditional practitioners into western-style medical institutions
proved more enduring, though there were resistances
and the mode of integration proved variable. In the
Hundred Flowers Campaign, one revealing article
observed that there were at least three ways in
which integration had been tried: (1) Traditional
doctors were integrated into all departments of
existing medical facilities. (2) Traditional doctors were given their own departments within western-
style institutions. (3) Traditional physicians were
given entirely separate facilities.[55] The author of
this article recommended that method number one
definitely be dropped; this became Ministry policy.

> Since the end of last year [1958], many hospi-
> tals have set up departments for traditional

114

Chinese medicine, and large numbers of hospitals and clinics of traditional Chinese medicine have been established.[56]

The integration approach, when carried to its most extreme lengths, called upon traditional practitioners to make daily rounds with their western-style colleagues. Interviews make it clear that there was an intangible quality of mutual respect in consultations which determined their actual content. Western-style doctors often did not respect traditional practitioners; they were aware of that and generally deferred.

We have seen a two-step process by which central policy was "distorted" during implementation.[57] Mao called for the "union" of the two schools, leaving it unclear what this meant in an operational sense. The Wei-sheng-pu adopted modes of integration which were least offensive to its constituency. Professionals rendered that still less effective by subtle modes of personal interaction.

Guidelines with regard to the establishment of separate Chung-i medical facilities proved more durable because at least the traditional medical community had some stake in their existence. In addition, their success was not so entirely dependent upon the cooperation of western-style personnel. The one likely source of friction would logically have been over the allocation of funds between western and Chinese-style institutions, but this is something about which we know nothing.

In December 1957, there were four colleges of traditional medicine. A year later, there were thirteen,[58] all of which had five-year curricula. The traditional physicians interviewed by Rifkin demonstrated pride in these schools.[59] Somewhat ironically, then, within a movement full of rhetoric deprecating professionals, policy was aimed at strengthening a profession.

As we have repeatedly noted, the eddies and flows of policy are complex, even within a single period. While the institutional position of Chung-i was being strengthened in the educational field, it was weakened on the research front. In 1955, the Academy of Traditional Medicine had been established and charged with three tasks: (1) Conduct research into Chinese drugs. (2) Coordinate all research relating to Chung-i. (3) Form a committee called the Chinese Medicine Research Committee (Chung-i Hsüeh-shu Yen-chiu Wei-yüan-hui) responsible for overseeing all Chung-i work.[60] During the Hundred

Flowers Campaign, medical professionals in the Ministry attacked the Chinese Medicine Research Committee for its failure to adequately perform the tasks assigned it; these individuals called for the Academy of Medical Sciences to take over the Committee's responsibilities. In March 1959, just as research was receiving new encouragement, this proposal was implemented, leaving the Academy of Traditional Medicine to write the history of Chinese medicine.[61]

While these policies were being implemented in the Ministry, traditional medicine was simultaneously being promoted by the Nine Man Sub-committee and by Party committees in the provinces, counties, and communes. In these contexts, the restraining influence of professionals was largely absent, and the degree of popularization was much greater.

> Outright folk medicine, simple popular remedies, and unlettered rustic practitioners, were very much in vogue. Even the disappointment with the celebrated tadpole experiment in early 1958--almost half of the women swallowing them as a test of their effectiveness in contraception became pregnant--failed to dampen enthusiasm for indigenous remedies.[62]

In this issue area we have seen how policy varied depending upon the institutional context in which each facet of it was made. Within the Ministry, policy regarding the research components reflected greater professional input than educational policy; this was the case, generally, as we have seen. Medical professionals could not prevent a mass movement aimed at getting them to study Chung-i, but they were strong enough to get policy modified. Still more clearly, medical researchers in the Ministry succeeded in stripping the Academy of Traditional Medicine of important responsibilities. In contrast, popularization of Chung-i in the rural areas proceeded rapidly, alienating both traditional practitioners and western-style doctors alike. In the rural context, the institutional strength of both western and Chinese-style medical communities was limited.

Policy regarding mass health campaigns was formulated in contexts entirely removed from the Ministry of Public Health. Meeting in March 1956, the Nine-Man Sub-committee had called for a seven-year plan to eradicate schistosomiasis. The reason for this initial "go-slow" approach was that several points were in dispute. The first problem concerned linking mass campaigns with technical organizations under the Wei-sheng-pu.[63] Secondly, experts argued that a higher level of agricultural mechanization was the prerequisite for overcoming parasitic diseases.[64] Finally, medical personnel felt that treatment should be conducted in modern and sufficiently equipped facilities.

But reactionary bourgeois academic "authorities" --and doctors deeply influenced by them--maintained that the countryside was not equipped for safe treatment and advocated that the emphasis should be on opening "regular" modern hospitals in the county towns in which the sick should stay for treatment.[65]

As the Center's attention shifted to rural areas, with Mao proclaiming that rural transformation was primary, the Nine Man Sub-committee began to attack "conservative" medical professionals with increasing frequency. In late 1957, the Sub-committee's Shanghai meeting was primarily devoted to overcoming the "sectarianism" of professionals.[66] In May 1958, Wei Wen-po made the final break with medical professionals, calling for the "basic elimination" of schistosomiasis.[67] In June and July, a meeting was held in Soochow at which doctors admitted that they had been too conservative.[68]
At each of these meetings local cadres claimed that his or her locality had succeeded in tasks which the "experts" had previously deemed impossible. On the basis of these reports, still higher goals were set. Mao was so impressed by Yukiang County's claim to have eliminated schistosomiasis that he wrote a poem entitled "Farewell to the God of Plagues."[69] A fever pitch was reached in November 1958 when the All China Conference on Parasitic Diseases was held in Shanghai. The meeting's resolution not only called for elimination of schistosomiasis within one year, but it also called for the eradication of four additional parasitic diseases.

The extent and scope of the work and the results so far achieved may be gauged from the proposal at the conference that we strive to achieve by next year the basic eradication of the five major parasitic diseases.[70]

Like a leading character in a Greek tragedy, this mobilization system had a tragic flaw; there

117

were no individuals charged with objectively evaluating the progress which was, or was not, being made.[71] One three-man team, for instance, claimed to have thoroughly examined 1,200 persons per day. In addition, later reports have confirmed refugee reports that diagnosing and treating large numbers of patients infected with parasitic diseases created strains on the county hospitals and produced drug shortages.[72] Finally, though there is little documentation, refugees report (and later journal articles tend to confirm)[73] that a substantial number of adverse antimony reactions occurred because of the lack of control over drug distribution and the large dosages administered. When in Shanghai (1976), I was told at a hospital affiliated with Shanghai First Medical School that, even now, overdoses of antimony create a significant number of heart problems.

The mass antiparasite campaign was the result of political and administrative pressures that generated a chain of rapidly escalating expectations. From 1955 on, especially in the wake of the Hundred Flowers Campaign, Mao pushed for concentrating on raising agricultural production and increasing the level of rural welfare. The Nine Man Sub-committee was one part of this response. By 1958, non-medical Party cadres dominated the entire Sub-committee apparatus. Party cadres at levels below the Sub-committee were worried about pleasing superiors; they were in a political structure which evaluated personnel in terms of "results." In addition, the problems which these mass campaigns created affected these cadres least. It was the hospitals and drug producers that first felt the pinch, and they could always be denounced as "rightists." Experts who questioned the claims were branded "conservatives." In the last months of 1958 and the first months of 1959, then, cadres were in a hermetically sealed self-reinforcing environment. The only effective brake on such a process was peasant alienation and financial insolvency.

SUMMARY

By March 1958, authority over different health issues was fragmented among three major institutions. The way in which issues were allocated to these "arenas" reflected the major concerns of various central leaders and the constituencies which these individuals de facto represented. Mao believed that

118

the tide of alienation could be stemmed and production increased by providing more welfare services; eradicating parasitic diseases was an important component of this program. The Nine Man Sub-committee's policies reflected the lack of professional input and the dominance of political cadres. The communes were similar.

While the perceived alienation of ruralites was Mao's central concern, other central leaders (e.g., Chou En-lai and Lu Ting-i) were relatively more responsive to the disquietude of the bureaucracies for which they were responsible. While we do not know precisely how the division of labor between the bureaucracy and Party organs was arrived at, it is clear that Lu Ting-i and Premier Chou tried to protect the Ministry's most valued policy areas; hospital administration, medical schools, and medical research. Because the Wei-sheng-pu was dominated by professionals and limited by money, policy change (in areas under its control) was relatively limited. There was no attempt to entitle more urbanites to "free" care; high-level research received a great deal of emphasis. Curricula in higher-level schools stayed about the same until lengthened in early 1959. Similarly, while Chung-i was popularized in rural areas, the movement was much more subdued in urban medical facilities. While the Chairman had called for the fusion of the two traditions, western-style doctors only studied it for short periods.

These findings have importance for our understanding of the Chinese policy-making system. Policy-making in China has been seen as a cyclical process in which policies tend to move in wave-like synchronization, reflecting uniform shifts in either capabilities, leadership composition, attitude, or shifting coalitions.[74] From this perspective, one would not expect to find policies which emphasize professionalism coexisting with those emphasizing the capabilities of the masses.[75] Such divergences, however, are precisely what were found. The explanation for this is that different political arenas (or institutions) are responsible for different issue areas. Each political arena is characterized by different inputs, participants, values, and resources. This would lead the analyst to suppose that conflict over where policy should be made is often as important as what policy ought to be.

Finally, cooptation of the Ministry leadership has been a continual process. Richard Lowenthal has described the dilemma quite accurately.[76] Any regime must create a specialized bureaucracy in

order to modernize. In doing this, however, one
necessarily creates bureaucratic constituencies
which resist any diminution of their authority. In
the process of building a functioning administrative
structure, Chinese health bureaucrats, originally
brought into the Ministry to exert control, have
come to share an increasingly broad range of values
with the professionals they were supposed to regulate. As we shall see in the next chapter, people
like Hsu Yun-pei, who had been brought to the Ministry in order to make the organization responsive to
the Party, began to pursue policies consistent with
the concerns of professionals in the 1960s. Also,
the Party apparatus, itself, has had to functionally specialize in order to exert some degree of
leadership over the Ministries. This has, in turn,
produced fragmentation of the leadership at one
higher level, with central leaders identifying with
that portion of the society or bureaucracy for which
they feel most responsible.

NOTES

1. For documentation on the Third Plenum see,
Documents of Chinese Communist Party Central Com-
mittee, September 1956-April 1969 (Hong Kong: Union
Research Institute, 1971), pp. 109-110; see also, Ho
Piao, "Tsai Ch'üan-kuo I-yüan Kung-tso Hui-i-shang
Te Pao-kao" [Report to the National Hospital Work
Conference], Hsin-hua Pan-yüeh-k'an [New China semi-
monthly], no. 128 (March 1958), pp. 143-148; see
also, Hsi Yeh-t'un, "Ch'üan-kuo I-yüan Kung-tso
Hui-i-shang Te Chung-ta I-i" [The great signifi-
cance of the National Hospital Work Conference],
I-hsüeh Shih Yü Pao-chien Tsu-chih [Medical history
and health organization], no. 1 (1958), pp. 23-24;
see also, Mao Tse-tung, "Tsai Pa-chieh San Chung
Ch'üan-hui-i-shang Te Chiang-hua" [Speech at the
Third Plenum of the Eighth Central Committee], Mao
Tse-tung Ssu-hsiang Wan-sui [Long live the thought
of Mao Tse-tung] (Peking: 1969), pp. 122-126.

2. Mao Tse-tung, "Tsai Nan-ning Hui-i-shang Te
Chiang-hua" [Speech at the Nanning Conference], Mao
Tse-tung Ssu-hsiang Wan-sui, pp. 145-154.

3. See Ho Piao and Hsi Yeh-t'un.

4. Ezra Vogel, Canton Under Communism (Cambridge:
Harvard University Press, 1969), p. 218.

5. Mao Tse-tung, "Tsai Nan-ning Hui-i-shang Te
Chiang-hua" [Speech at the Nanning Conference], Mao
Tse-tung Ssu-hsiang Wan-sui, p. 151.

6. Hsi Yeh-t'un, p. 24.

7. Hsi Yeh-t'un, p. 23.

8. Mao Tse-tung, "Tsai Nan-ning Hui-i-shang Te
Chiang-hua" [Speech at the Nanning Conference], Mao
Tse-tung Ssu-hsiang Wan-sui, p. 153.

9. Li Teh-ch'uan, "Placing Health Undertakings at
the Service of Production," New China News Agency
(hereafter NCNA), April 27, 1959, in Current Background (hereafter CB), no. 577, p. 20; see also,
Li Teh-ch'uan, "Ten Years of Public Health Work in
New China," Chinese Medical Journal 79 (1959):486;
see also, Chu-yuan Cheng, "Health Manpower in Communist China" (Presented at the Macy Conference on
Public Health in the People's Republic of China,
Ann Arbor, Michigan, May 14-17, 1972), p. 17.

10. Cheng, p. 17; see also, Hsu Yun-pei, "Advance
the Great Work of Protecting the People's Health,"
Chinese Medical Journal 80 (1960):406.

11. "Thoroughly Criticize and Repudiate the Eight-
Year Medical Education Program Pushed by China's
Krushchev," China's Medicine 3 (1968):164-169.

12. Ezra Vogel, Interview No. 21, p. 1.

13. Mao Tse-tung, "Ho Ko Hsieh-tso Ch'ü Chu-jen Te
T'an-hua" [Talks with the leaders of various cooperative areas] (December 12, 1958), Mao Tse-tung Ssu-
hsiang Wan-sui, p. 257.

14. Mao Tse-tung, "Tsai Pa-chieh Liu Chung Ch'üan-
hui-i-shang Te Chiang-hua" [Speech to the Sixth
Plenum of the Eighth Central Committee], Mao Tse-
tung Ssu-hsiang Wan-sui, pp. 259-269.

15. Mao Tse-tung, "Ho Ko Hsieh-tso Ch'ü Chu-jen Te
T'an-hua" [Talks with the leaders of various cooperative areas], Mao Tse-tung Ssu-hsiang Wan-sui, p.
252.

16. Chou En-lai, "Report on Government Work," NCNA,
April 18, 1959, in CB, no. 559, pp. 16-17.

17. Li Huei-han, "Prevention and Treatment of Filariasis in Shantung Province," Chinese Medical Journal 78 (1959):54.

18. "The Orientation of the Revolution in Medical Education as Seen in the Growth of 'Barefoot Doctors'," China's Medicine 10 (1968):574.

19. "Thoroughly Criticize and Repudiate," pp. 164-165.

20. "Thoroughly Criticize and Repudiate," p. 165. Interestingly, Lu-Ting-i had studied in the United States.

21. David M. Lampton, "Health Policy During the Great Leap Forward," China Quarterly (hereafter CQ), no. 60 (1974), pp. 672-673.

22. "Chung-i Yan-chiu Kung-tso-chung Te Chi-ko Wen-t'i" [A few problems in the research of Chinese medicine], Chien-k'ang Pao [Health bulletin], January 29, 1957.

23. Jen-min Jih-pao [People's daily], March 10, 1959.

24. Joshua Horn, Away With All Pests (New York: Monthly Review Press, 1969), Chapter 11.

25. Li Teh-ch'uan, "Placing Health Undertakings at the Service of Production," NCNA, April 27, 1959, in CB, no. 577, p. 20. This speech was delivered at the First Session of the Second National People's Congress.

26. David M. Lampton, Interview File 21 E, no. 3, p. 3.

27. Chou En-lai, "Report on Government Work," p. 17.

28. "Sectional Medical Service Adopted in Over Thirty Cities," Jen-min Jih-pao [People's daily], October 22, 1957, in Survey of the China Mainland Press (hereafter SCMP), no. 1645, pp. 19-20; see also, Ezra Vogel, Interview No. 2, p. 1.

29. David M. Lampton, Interview File 21 E.

30. Li Teh-ch'uan, "Placing Health Undertakings at the Service of Production," p. 19.

31. "China's Health Work in the Past Decade," NCNA, September 20, 1959, CB, no. 609, p. 42.

32. It is difficult to know what this precisely means. Were all drugs reduced 34 percent or was this an average? If it is an average, which drugs were reduced more and which less?

33. "Pharmaceuticals in New China," Chinese Medical Journal 80 (1960):208.

34. David M. Lampton, Interview File 21 E.

35. "Pharmaceuticals in New China," p. 208.

36. Michel Oksenberg, Interview No. 2, p. 1.

37. Ezra Vogel, Interview No. 30, p. 5.

38. Ezra Vogel, Interview No. 30, p. 5.

39. "An Investigation Report on How the Ch'ünhsing Brigade in Ch'üchiang Hsien, Kwangtung Province Firmly Adheres to Cooperative Medical Service Over the Past Eleven Years," Hung Ch'i [Red flag], no. 1 (1969), in Selections from China Mainland Magazines (hereafter SCMM), no. 642, p. 28; see also, Jen-min Jih-pao [People's daily], December 7, 1968.

40. "Cooperative Medical System Introduced in Honan," Jen-min Jih-pao [People's daily], September 24, 1958, in SCMP, no. 1871, p. 31.

41. "An Investigation Report on How the Ch'ün-hsing . . .", p. 32.

42. Audrey Donnithorne, China's Economic System (New York: Praeger, 1967), p. 72.

43. "An Investigation Report on How the Ch'ün-hsing . . .", p. 28.

44. One respondent described how county hospital costs grew. ". . . his patients were mostly farmers or cadres. The latter had their medical bills paid by the Government, whereas the former had to pay their own. Sometimes the farmers did not have the money to pay for the treatment, but the doctors would give him [sic] everything he needed, even though they knew they would not be paid." Ezra Vogel, Interview No. 13, p. 5.

45. Nai-ruenn Chen, Chinese Economic Statistics (Chicago: Aldine, 1967), p. 446; see also, Li Hsien-nien, "Report on Final State Accounts, 1958 and the Draft State Budget 1959," NCNA, April 21, 1959, in CB, no. 562, pp. 1-9.

46. Nai-ruenn Chen, p. 446.

47. Roderick MacFarquhar, The Origins of the Cultural Revolution, Vol. I (New York: Columbia University Press, 1974), pp. 68-74.

48. David M. Lampton, Interview File 21 E.

49. John W. Lewis, Leadership in Communist China (Ithaca: Cornell University Press, 1963), pp. 110-111. Lewis notes that while Party membership grew from 12.72 million in 1957 to 13.96 million in 1959, much of this increase may have been the result of the Party's need to increase cadre strength in the people's communes.

50. Ezra Vogel, Interview No. 21, p. 1.

51. "Earnest Implementation of the Party's Policy on Traditional Chinese Medicine," Chinese Medical Journal 78 (1959):205-206.

52. "Earnest Implementation of the Party's Policy on Traditional Chinese Medicine," p. 209.

53. Chou En-lai, "Report on Government Work," CB, no. 559, p. 17.

54. Hei-lung-kiang Jih-pao [Heilungkiang daily], June 7, 1957.

55. "Kuan-yü Chung-i Ts'an-chia I-yüan Kung-tso Te Chi-ko Wen-t'i" [Several problems regarding the participation of traditional practitioners in hospital work], Chien-k'ang Pao [Health bulletin], March 11, 1957.

56. "News and Notes," Chinese Medical Journal 79 (1959):479.

57. Jeffrey Pressman and Aaron Wildavsky, Implementation (Berkeley: University of California Press, 1974). This study describes the difficulties in achieving policy objectives even if implementing agencies share the goals of central policy-makers.

58. "Recent Achievements in the Promotion of Traditional Chinese Medicine," Chinese Medical Journal 78 (1959):105; see also, Chinese Medical Journal 75 (1957):956.

59. Susan Rifkin, Interviews With Traditional Doctors. I would like to thank Ms. Rifkin for making these protocols available.

60. "Chung-i Yan-chiu Kung-tso-chung Te Chi-ko Went'i" [A few problems in the research of traditional Chinese medicine], Chien-k'ang Pao [Health bulletin], January 25, 1957.

61. "I-hsüeh K'o-hsüeh-yüan Ho Chung-i Yan-chiu-yüan Ta Hsieh-tso" [The cooperation of the Academy of Medical Sciences and the Academy of Traditional Medicine], Jen-min Jih-pao [People's daily], March 10, 1959.

62. Ralph Croizier, Traditional Medicine in Modern China (Cambridge: Harvard University Press, 1968), p. 187.

63. "Wei-sheng Fang-i-chan Ho Ai-kuo Wei-sheng Yün-tung Wei-yüan-hui Tsen-yang P'ei-ho?" [How can health prevention stations and patriotic health campaigns be integrated?], Chien-k'ang Pao [Health bulletin] January 18, 1957.

64. Wen-hui Pao, September 29, 1958.

65. "A Great Victory of Mao Tse-tung's Thought in the Battle Against Schistosomiasis," China's Medicine, no. 10 (1968), p. 594.

66. Wen-hui Pao, December 11, 1957.

67. Jen-min Jih-pao [People's daily], May 16, 1958.

68. Kuang-ming Jih-pao [Bright daily], July 6, 1958.

69. Jerome Ch'ên, Mao and the Chinese Revolution (London: Oxford University Press, 1965), p. 349.

70. "All China Conference on Parasitic Diseases," Chinese Medical Journal 77 (1958):519.

71. Even the usually cautious "tide watcher," Chou En-lai, is alleged to have said in September 1958, "Smash the bourgeois medical powers and establish

the proletarian spirit." Ch'üan-wu-ti [Invincible],
no. 17, p. 3.

72. Hangchow Chekiang Provincial Service in Mandarin, February 27, 1974, Foreign Broadcast Information Service: Daily Report, People's Republic of
China, no. 53 (1974), p. C3.

73. "Manufacture and Clinical Application of Cardiac Pacemaker," Chinese Medical Journal, no. 1
(1974), p. 1. This article noted that high doses of
antimony could produce heart problems.

74. G. William Skinner and Edwin Winckler, "Com-
pliance Succession in Rural Communist China: A
Cyclical Theory," in A Sociological Reader on Com-
plex Organizations, ed. Amitai Etzioni (New York:
Holt, Rinehart and Winston, 1969), pp. 410-438;
see also, Parris H. Chang, Power and Policy in China
(University Park: Pennsylvania State University
Press, 1975).

75. This case is argued in more detail in David
M. Lampton, "Health Policy During the Great Leap
Forward."

76. Richard Lowenthal, "Development vs. Utopia in
Communist Policy," in Change in Communist Systems,
ed. Chalmers Johnson (Stanford: Stanford University
Press, 1970), pp. 33-116.

PART 3

THE COLLAPSE OF THE
GREAT LEAP FORWARD:
TOWARD THE FRAGMENTATION
OF LEADERSHIP

Chapter 6
ON DOMINOES: ONE STEP BACK FROM THE GREAT LEAP FORWARD (1960-1965)

<u>INTRODUCTION</u>

The principal organizational and political fact of the Great Leap Forward was that there had been a proliferation of arenas in which policy (of every kind) was made. This made it difficult to achieve program coordination, even when it was essential. The absolute precondition for the success of programs coming from the communes and the Nine Man Subcommittee was the rapid expansion of agricultural production. Increased agricultural output was essential in order to finance new rural programs and to maintain peasant morale. By 1959, however, it was clear that decreases in agricultural production were imminent and that, before long, these declines would reverberate throughout the industrial and urban sectors of the economy.

According to almost all estimates, including those of the Chinese, agricultural production declined, with all but the Chinese agreeing that the decline began in 1959.[1] In 1959, according to the estimates of the United States Consulate General in Hong Kong, the decline in grain output between 1958 and 1960 was 18 percent.[2] Other estimates indicate that far more substantial declines may have occurred.[3] By 1960, the reduction in rural demand, and the concurrent shortage of raw materials for industry, precipitated declines in industrial output in 1960 and 1961, according to Field's estimates.[4] As would be expected, declines in agricultural and industrial output necessitated reduction in both imports and exports in the 1960-1962 period.[5] The need to import grain in the face of a shrinking total value of foreign trade meant that the importation of capital goods was exceedingly limited; this retarded long-term economic expansion further.

These tremendous economic difficulties had political repercussions, the most conspicuous of which was the torrent of approximately 142,000 refugees which poured into Hong Kong in 1962.[6] The domestic food situation in 1961 was so precarious that the Rear Services Department of the Mukden Military Region reported that a major campaign to obtain "food substitutes" was under way.

> . . . there were 1,808 animals of various kinds caught. . . . In December alone there were collected over 28,000,000 catties of various kinds of materials [for food]. By the end of December 2,500,000 catties of artificial glutenous [sic. glutinous] flour, 2,910 catties of artificial meat essence, 7,709 catties of 'lien-pao-mei' [a kind of fungus], and 5,605 catties of albumen were made.[7]

Also, as the economic situation decayed, rural speculation and other unsanctioned practices became increasingly widespread.

The Ministry of Public Health and its subordinate hospitals, as well as the Nine Man Sub-committee and commune health programs, could not remain insulated from economic and political disruption of such proportions. In the next two chapters we shall demonstrate that health care action policy in the 1960-1965 period reflected the differential ability of the Wei-sheng-pu leadership to move ahead in its policy areas and the inability of the Nine Man Sub-committee and the Commune Party Committees to move ahead in the areas for which they had responsibility. The argument is that the foundations upon which the Great Leap had been built were washed out by economic dislocations and the resulting elite and social fragmentation. In essence, the Leap had avoided hard allocation decisions by attempting to give everyone what they wanted. This was a viable strategy as long as the economy generated the resources. Once the illusion of plenty had been shattered, however, the mass campaigns and communes were the most immediately and adversely affected. They were the most dependent on peasant morale and rising agricultural production.

CONTINUITY AND CHANGE IN RETRENCHMENT LEADERSHIP

Important changes in leadership occurred in each of the three major health policy-making forums. Regarding the Sub-committee, as noted, the high-tide of the Great Leap Forward had considerably diminished

130

the role of medical professionals. Party zealots, especially at the middle levels, were locked into a system in which overoptimistic leadership goals produced exaggerated cadre claims, which further escalated leadership expectations. Early in 1960, this process began to reverse as two things occurred: First, the Sub-committee (once again) sought expert advice.[8] In announcing a Sub-committee meeting in July 1960, it was revealed that Vice-Minister of Public Health Ch'ien Hsin-chung had spoken. The sense of the meeting was that research in parasitic diseases should, once again, be undertaken. Ch'ien had been identified with basic medical research for years and the Sub-committee's new emphasis seems to reflect his input. Signalling the new trend, Red Flag carried an article by Vice-Minister of Health Ho Piao in which the doctor said,

> The present picture of rural health work is good, but, to accomplish the great and diffi-cult task of elimination of diseases, long-term persistent effort is needed.[9] (emphasis added).

Ho was saying what was now apparent to all; there were no shortcuts.

Secondly, within the Sub-committee, there was an apparent deterioration of support for the contin-uation of mass campaigns. While knowing little about intracommittee dynamics, we do know that Sub-committee member Liao Lu-yen was minister of agri-culture and deputy director of the Party Rural Work Department. Mao subsequently rebuked that depart-ment for its opposition to his rural mobilizational policies.[10] Oksenberg has noted that Teng Tzu-hui and Liao Lu-yen were, in effect, "brokers" for peasant discontent.[11] Irrespective of whether or not they were brokers, and regardless of what their initial position on mass campaigns had been, once agricultural production sagged in 1959 and 1960, there was a symmetry of interest between their need to increase production and the manifest desire of the peasants for a relaxation of mobilization. Similarly, one would expect that Hsu Yun-pei would have reflected the Wei-sheng-pu's discontent to the Sub-committee.

Reflective of both the expert input and the loss of internal Sub-committee cohesion was the fact that after July 1960, the Sub-committee held no further publicly announced sessions until January 1964.[12] The fact that the Sub-committee ceased making policy is related, at least chronologically,

to the beginning of Mao's "retreat to the second
line of leadership." Mao had given up the presi-
dency in 1958, though he continued to exercise an
important role in rectification work until at least
the Tenth Plenum of September 1962. In health policy, the documentary history supports the proposition
that Mao lost influence (or lost interest) rather
rapidly. Mao made no statements on health care
after July 20, 1960. In two speeches (March and
April 1960),[13] Mao called for more mass campaigns.
After the July 11-20, 1960 Standing Committee
meeting of the Sub-committee, which firmly rejected
further mass campaigns, Mao was silent on health
policy until January 1964, when he made a cryptic
comment about his doctor;[14] only in August 1964 did
he blast medical policy.[15]

In short, the national leadership of mass campaign work changed in three ways: (1) Experts
played an augmented role and pushed for more
research. (2) Sub-committee members were no longer
willing to support Mao's call for such campaigns.
(3) Mao discontinued playing an active role in articulating health policy.

The communes. Momentous changes occurred in
commune leadership during this period. In May
1961, new "draft" regulations (The Sixty Articles)
were issued which effectively cut the size of the
average commune by two-thirds.

> The scale of the people's commune at the vari-
> ous levels should in every case be such as to
> benefit production, operation and management,
> and organizational life, and ought not to be
> excessively large. . . . In general, the
> people's commune should be equivalent in scale
> to the original hsiang or large hsiang.[16]

This meant that China was reducing commune size so
that it would be roughly equivalent to the old upper-
level agricultural producers' cooperative. This
reestablished rough alignment with traditional
standard marketing areas.

These administrative gymnastics are important
because they give us a hint as to who the new
leaders of communes (and commune health centers)
were and what level of organization was feasible.
These administrative alterations changed the locus
of control over the rural health system and changed
the size of the covered population. Cadres lower in
the rural hierarchy, along with practitioners in

132

"united clinics," became the leaders of what rural
health system there was.

Cadres at the multi-<u>hsiang</u> level (the 1958-1959
commune) lost control for two clusters of reasons.
They no longer had organizational roles when the size
of the commune unit was reduced by two-thirds.
Simultaneously, leadership at lower levels (the
<u>hsiang</u> and village) played an increasingly active
part; this leadership stratum had many more ties
(familial, friendship, and economic) with the surrounding peasants than the previous commune leadership had had. Also, within these smaller communes,
the "basic accounting unit" (<u>chi-pen kwai-chi dan-
wei</u>) was successively moved from the commune, to the
production brigade, to the production team.[17] Again,
cadres with strong local ties gained authority.

> . . . the income of the lower rural cadres is
> directly linked with the incomes of the peas-
> ants. . . . It can be seen that a significant
> dividing line runs between those who are "state
> cadres" and who look to higher rungs of Party
> and state hierarchies for the approbation which
> can further their careers and the lower cadres
> who are first and foremost local peasants,
> subject to the pressures from their fellows.
> The decentralization of authority from the com-
> mune to the production team between 1958 and
> 1962 effected a transfer of power to those
> cadres most nearly identified with local
> people.[18]

In short, by breaking up the large communes and then
transferring fiscal and planning authority downward,
the leaders making decisions about rural health care
had changed, the resources available to them had
diminished, and the size of the population for which
they had responsibility was reduced.

<u>The Ministry of Public Health's leadership</u>
underwent minor alterations. There were only three
changes of personnel at the vice-ministerial level.
One of these was necessary due to the death of
Vice-Minister Su Ching-kuan.[19] Su had been the
first western-style physician to join the Red Army
and had been in the <u>Wei-sheng-pu</u> since liberation.

With Su's death in 1964, Shih Shu-han became
vice-minister of health the following year. Shih
had been the deputy director of public health in
the Northwest Military and Administrative Region
in the early 1950s, and had medical training.
Shih's wife, Fan K'un-hsien, worked in Peking

Hospital,[20] as did Shen Yu-ts'un, the wife of Ch'ien Hsin-chung.[21] One would expect that Ministry leaders with both medical training themselves and relatives practicing in elite hospitals would be relatively responsive to the professional dissatisfactions that arose during the 1960s.

The second leadership change occurred when Wu Yun-fu was transferred to the Party Control Commission in April 1963.[22] As far as we know, Wu had no medical background (he had worked with organizations such as the Red Cross). His transfer would seem to have had the effect of at least diminishing the numerical strength of nonprofessionals in the councils of the Ministry.

The remaining Ministry appointee was Kuo Tzu-hua who apparently took charge of the Bureau of Traditional Medicine (Chung-i-ssu) in July 1961. Kuo had been Minister Li Teh-ch'uan's assistant since the mid-1950s. While we do not know his professional background, he did promote policies which assuaged the fears of both traditional and western-style doctors; he greatly reduced the popularization of Chung-i.[23] Additionally, he emphasized research (with which everyone could agree) and more thorough traditional education.

Perhaps the most important (and least observable) aspect of leadership change was the cooptation of Hsu Yun-pei and Chang Kai and the increasing influence of medically expert vice-ministers within the Ministry of Public Health.[24] While speculative, it appears that the Great Leap had weakened the position of those vice-ministers who had been closely identified with the excesses of Leap policies (e.g., Hsu Yun-pei who had been on the Subcommittee). Cultural Revolution documents assert that both Hsu and Chang Kai became increasingly articulate spokesmen for professionally approved policies.[25] One could hypothesize that this represented Hsu and Chang's attempt to maintain some degree of influence over the organization. Irrespective of the validity of this, Ch'ien Hsin-chung, not First Vice-Minister Hsu, was named Minister of Health in early 1965, upon the retirement of Li Teh-ch'uan.

Not only did the locus of decision-making authority within the Wei-sheng-pu shift, but so did authority in the multitude of hospitals and research centers dotting the landscape. Decision-making became much more consultative. Doctors became the de facto heads of hospitals, with political cadres oftentimes playing ceremonial roles.[26]

In all spheres, the effect of retrenchment was to raise the status of older and more experienced personnel even if they had been accused of having bourgeois tendencies.[27]

In sum, the health system's leadership changed in three ways: Personnel switches were made, alterations in elite attitudes appeared to have occurred, and a shift in effective authority within the Wei-sheng-pu's leadership took place. Within medical facilities, decision-making became more consultative, with doctors exercising greater influence.

LEADERSHIP'S EVALUATION OF THE PROBLEMS

The Nine Man Sub-committee on Schistosomiasis faced a complex situation in which there was a substantial reduction in grain production, leading to peasant alienation.[28] The first problem was that peasants became increasingly less willing to be mobilized for mass health campaigns. At the same time, the objective measures of health were declining.[29]

If you set foot in the major streets or side alleys of this ancient townlet, you can find animals such as pigs, chickens and dogs moving about freely in the street or discharging urine and dung everywhere.[30]

While the Sub-committee was faced with these health problems, local cadres were either unable, or unwilling, to mobilize the population.

A great number of rural residents in Ch'inhsien, Linghsien, and other hsien are also stricken with the hookworm disease. This shows that our cadres have not paid adequate attention to the matter and made no earnest efforts to stamp out thoroughly the diseases. . . . We believe that apart from the fact that the leading cadres at the hsien and commune levels are indifferent to the suffering of the masses from disease, the Provincial Health Department should bear the great part of the responsibility.[31]

A more reasonable hypothesis concerning the origins of cadre unwillingness to mobilize the populace is that they were extremely sensitive to "the suffering of the masses." Local cadres knew all too well that

135

peasants were generally unwilling to submit to any more mass campaigns when production was declining and their standard of living deteriorating.

The reduction in commune size, along with the designation of the production team as the "basic accounting unit," meant that there was no unit of rural organization with sufficient powers (over a wide enough area) to make mass campaigns feasible. In addition, low-level decision-making tended to exaggerate the importance of economic considerations and diminish the potency of ideological factors. After all, teams had been designated the basic accounting unit precisely because they emphasized production. The creation of private plots further diminished the incentive to spend time on mass campaigns.

The Sub-committee was not only constrained by problems at the basic level, changes in attitude and influence at the Party Center were important as well. In 1959 and 1960, leadership solidarity was breaking down over a wide range of issues. The dismissal of P'eng Teh-huai, who called the Great Leap Forward "petty-bourgeois fanaticism," was the most dramatic manifestation of this fact.[32] Subsequently, in the 1961-1962 period, writers with high-level political connections, men like Wu Han, T'ien Han, and Teng T'o, all criticized Chairman Mao for the excesses of the Leap.[33]

Specific issues were also apparently a source of conflict. In January 1960, Mao is reported to have said, ". . . we ought not promote awards of merit, Ph.D.'s and this sort of thing." Liu Shao-ch'i is said to have responded that "whether or not degrees should be promoted or not is worth investigating." Teng Hsiao-p'ing is accused of blatantly directing lower levels "to quickly write a report on this and send it up, approved . . . and don't only promote doctors and Academy personnel and engineers. . . ." Vice-Minister of Public Health Ch'ien Hsin-chung agreed saying, "Degrees are international, we must not lightly deny them."[34]

By 1961, Mao was faced with leadership division and he had two options: fight it out then and there (in the face of economic decline and social dissatisfactions) or concentrate on a limited range of issues, like rectification and international affairs, which were not so divisive. By narrowing his concerns he could focus his energies. He adopted the latter strategy.

As to the question of unity within the Party. Unity of the Central Committee is the heart of

136

> the unity of the whole Party. At the Lushan
> Conference, there was a small number of people
> who were opposed to unity, [but] we must pro-
> ceed toward unity. Making progress is well and
> good, but are we really making progress? They
> say: "You have made mistakes too!" This is
> right . . . the Center and the localities have
> all made mistakes.[35]

In the context of 1960-1961, promoting unity could
only mean putting the brakes on mobilization in the
countryside. Whether Mao really favored this policy,
or merely acquiesced to something with which he was
fundamentally opposed, is something we may never
know.

The problems confronting the rural leadership.
The difficulties facing the commune, brigade, and
team leaders were numerous. Commune, brigade, and
team welfare funds were reduced in size. As a consequence, less money was available for subsidized
(or "free") medical treatment at any level in the
communes.[36] Secondly, not only were funds scarce,
more people were sick. Per capita health demands
were escalating in the face of declining revenues.
For instance, Ch'ünhsing Brigade in Ch'üchiang
County, Kwangtung, reported that a "seriously ill"
woman and her children had cost the cooperative
medical service 970 yüan (hereafter ¥). Assuming
that three individuals were involved, this was a per
capita cost of slightly more than 320¥. This report
went on to note that 2 percent of the brigade's population had been "seriously ill" (58 persons).[37] If
the cost was the same for each "seriously ill" individual, that would have required an outlay in excess
of 18,500¥. Judging from the size of other welfare
funds, Ch'ünhsing's welfare fund was probably nowhere near that size. This suggests that many commune health programs were basically insolvent without outside subsidy.

Further compounding the difficulties facing
local cadres, food production had fallen so substantially that acreage previously devoted to growing
medicinal herbs had to be converted to grain production.[38] This meant that rural traditional practitioners faced drug shortages and the consumer
was forced to pay more for traditional pharmaceuticals. Vice-Minister Ho Piao specifically noted,
"The production of Chinese medical material should
be combined with reforestation as much as possible
to minimize the taking up of arable land."[39]

Local cadres faced intracommune political divisions as well. Brigade cadres, for example, often

137

wanted to keep control of brigade industries so they would have a larger financial base. On the other hand, team leaders found it in their interest to secure control of these enterprises.[40] Similarly, wealthy teams and brigades wanted to eliminate commune or brigade health programs because they were, in effect, subsidizing less prosperous units. In short, there were internal commune political pressures pushing for an elimination of redistributive programs. These forces demanded decentralization of commune economic control which made locally supported rural welfare programs almost impossible at this time.

In addition, national directives called for elimination of all programs which had an adverse impact on agricultural production. The most important of these regulations was the "Sixty Articles." One PLA directive commenting on this document noted,

> Problems existing in the work of communes, especially the problem of two equalizations, must be seriously and carefully overcome. We have always opposed equalization, for it denies the difference in income and distribution between [production] teams and between commune members. And the denial of this distinction is a denial of the Socialist principle "to each according to his work, and the more work the more pay."[41]

The regulations making the production team the basic accounting unit administered the coup de grâce to comprehensive commune health care. Production teams were far too small to run a solvent health care system, and brigades and communes had been denied the revenues to do so.

In short, the local cadre was presented with an entire galaxy of difficulties. First, the optimal unit for increasing production was the team; this was not the optimal unit for health care administration. Secondly, political pressures within the commune resisted redistributive programs. Finally, central directives emphasized production.

The Wei-sheng-pu's definition of the situation. The one overwhelming problem facing the Ministry of Public Health was, how could county and major urban hospitals cope with the flood of patients? This basic problem broke down into a series of subsidiary hurdles. How could staffs be trained, facilities expanded, and sufficient equipment and drugs obtained? The Ministry faced many of the same problems it

138

always had, though the context was somewhat different. The description provided by one interviewee
provides part of that context.

> After the failure of the Great Leap Forward,
> there were so many people seeking health care,
> even in the cities, that long lines formed at
> XX hospital and that if you wanted attention
> the next day you would take warm belongings and
> queue up the night before. Also, . . . it was
> not uncommon for those who were well to queue
> up the night before and then when the very sick
> came in the morning to be at the end of the line
> and so desperate that they would buy places at
> the front of the line for $1. . . .[42]

The second problem confronting Ministry and
hospital administrators was a breakdown in the authority structure within many medical facilities.
Doctors and professional staff were highly dissatisfied; one of the most influential leaders of the
Chinese Medical Association said that such chaos
would never happen again, if he could help it.[43]
These difficulties inspired Bright Daily to write
an article entitled, "To Fix the Responsibilities
and Duties of Doctors and Nurses; To Perfect Regulations and Systems."[44]

While physicians, in their clinical roles, had
been the most disturbed during the Leap, even
research had not been entirely insulated. Doctors
often had both clinical and research responsibilities; turbulence in one area spilled over into the
other. T'ao Chu sarcastically indicated that during
the Leap conditions for research had been far from
optimal.

> Conditions are required for scientific research.
> They are required even for hair-dressing. At
> least there must be a barber's shop. They are
> more necessary in scientific research. One,
> conditions are necessary; two, assistants are
> necessary; three, data are necessary; four,
> certain material supplies are necessary.[45]

Perhaps the most important difficulty was
sagging revenues. The one available source on the
Chinese budget for this period indicates that actual
revenues in the 1960-1964 period dropped to about
50 percent of the budgeted levels.[46] While we do
not know exactly, one would expect that the Ministry
would have been hurt at least in rough proportion to
the total decline in available resources.

Sagging revenues hit provincial and county governments as well. Because the Wei-sheng-pu's past strategy had been to give local health bureaus as many tasks as possible, when local revenues declined substantially, many of these duties could no longer be performed. This led, as we shall see, to the closure of many middle-level medical schools. Because central resources were simultaneously declining, the Ministry was less able to provide subsidies. One would anticipate that regional disparities in the provision of health services grew, reflecting the differential impact of agricultural declines, though we have no data on this point.

The final major difficulty concerned the decline in drug quality and reliability. Doctors, patients, large pharmaceutical manufacturers, and the staff of the Ministry's Bureau of Drugs (Yao-cheng-chü) were all unhappy about declines in quality.[47] From their viewpoint, solving the problem required increased investment in the pharmaceutical industry, more efficient management of existing facilities, elimination and consolidation of small producers, reduction in waste of already manufactured drugs, and increased quality control.

LEADERSHIP RESOURCES

Subsequent action policies reflected the fact that not all three policy-making arenas were hit in the same way by post-Leap changes in the resource base. In fact, it was the differential impact of resource declines which helps explain why some policy areas changed little and others more drastically.

The Nine Man Sub-committee. The economic, social, and political resources of the Sub-committee all changed rapidly in 1960. First of all, the "Sixty Articles," and the subsequent devolution of rural power to the production teams, meant that there was no longer an organizational structure capable of mobilizing the peasants. Secondly, because increasing agricultural production was the immediate need, both the government and the peasantry agreed about one thing: nothing should interfere with the drive to increase production. In the short-run, mass mobilization could be nothing but counterproductive to that effort.

Not only did economic and structural considerations weaken the Sub-committee, but so did changes in political relations at both the Center and within

140

the Sub-committee itself. While information is
scant, it appears that members of the Sub-committee
were caught in a web of contradictory loyalties.
Knowing the past opposition of Ministry personnel
to the mass campaigns, one can conjecture that Hsu
Yun-pei was continually subjected to the professional pressures emanating from the organization for
which he was responsible. Similarly, Liao Lu-yen,
as the Minister of Agriculture, was responsible for
increasing agricultural production. When his duties
on the Sub-committee conflicted with those as Minister, he appears to have chosen to emphasize production.[48] In short, not only had the political situation in the countryside altered, it had also changed
within the Sub-committee.

Political relationships at the Center changed
as well. Mao lost ground to more bureaucratically
oriented leaders like Chou En-lai, Liu Shao-ch'i,
Teng Hsiao-p'ing, and P'eng Chen (then First Party
Secretary of Peking and member of the Politburo).
Earlier we noted that Mao's preferences vis à vis
mass campaigns and medical education either had been
partially or wholly rejected. Mao, himself, said
that Teng Hsiao-p'ing and Liu Shao-ch'i ignored him
after 1959. The Chairman asserted that both men
treated him,

> . . . like their dead parent at a funeral. When
> we had a meeting, Teng Hsiao-p'ing always sat
> in the place furthest away from me. Since 1959
> he has not briefed me on the work of the Cen-
> tral Committee Secretariat.[49]

It appears, then, that while the Sub-committee was
fragmenting, Mao was losing his capacity to provide
the momentum necessary to continue Sub-committee
work; Mao's priorities may have changed as well.
Both of these trends were intimately tied to the
deteriorating rural situation.

The communes. The political and economic
resources of cadres at the commune and brigade levels
were even more dismal.

> The higher authorities tried to shift on to the
> lower cadres much of the blame for the agricul-
> tural disasters of the post-1958 period. Con-
> sequently the cadres felt themselves ground
> between unreasonable superiors and a discon-
> tented peasantry and their resentment bred
> listlessness. The cadres of production bri-
> gades, in particular, felt that their position

had been undermined by the devolution of power to the teams. "Now that production brigades have been deprived even of the authority over production and distribution, . . . what should we do if a production team does not listen to us?" . . . "When there is no rice in your hands, not even the chickens will come to you."[50]

One manifestation of these declines in commune and brigade economic resources (a decrease which we have already analyzed) was the reduction in the number of rural health workers. The total pool of health personnel fell from 2.16 million in 1958, to 1.94 million in 1961, to 1.4 million in 1963.[51] Most of this reduction occurred among local and para-medic personnel. Yukiang County, Kiangsu, for instance, had 3,900 health workers in 2,500 production brigades in June 1960. Subsequently, this number was reduced to 300.[52] Neither brigades nor communes had the resources to support these personnel, and teams were not large enough to effectively do so, even if they had wanted to.

In weighing whether or not to allocate scarce funds to health care, commune leaders at all levels had to ask, can these personnel perform tasks which justify the expenditures? Even assuming that commune health personnel were highly competent (and there is no reason to assume this was uniformly the case), with no drugs or equipment, with tighter requirements that communes pay for people referred to urban facilities, and with the utility of each yüan increasing, cooperative health care just does not appear to have been a high priority. In making the production team the basic accounting unit, the Center faced this dilemma: How can we progress toward agrarian socialism, which rests upon a foundation of "plenty," when the only means by which that "plenty" can be achieved are fundamentally anti-socialist?

The Wei-sheng-pu's resources did not uniformly rise or fall during this period; one has to analyze each resource separately. The biggest asset the Ministry had was the potential cooperation of almost every sector of Chinese society in trying to upgrade the urban hospital system. First of all, both patients and doctors felt they had suffered as a consequence of the Leap; doctors because they had not been able to provide the care that they thought they should and patients because they had not received it.[53] Party cadres and insured workers were especially adamant about this. Similarly, city

142

leaders like Peking's P'eng Chen felt that the Leap had precipitated a decline in urban conditions; they pushed for placing emphasis on urban areas.[54] Finally, even peasants acquiesced (if they had any influence at all). Care at the county hospital was the only alternative to none at all.

The Wei-sheng-pu's ability to gain the compliance of doctors, researchers, and medical professors went up once the Party's policy of support for experts was unambiguously given. While policy toward experts had started to shift as early as 1959, by the end of 1961, the signs of central encouragement were everywhere. In September, T'ao Chu made a "Report to Higher Intellectuals" in which he said,

> . . . the Party's leadership must be free from formalism. Party leadership requires making friends and rallying all round the Party. Party leadership does not gain strength by holding numerous meetings or talking about empty principles.[55]

At the same time, Ch'en I made similar remarks to physicians in Canton.[56] By December, Red Flag had given its blessings to the policy.[57] The Ministry could unabashedly use technical personnel.

By all accounts, money was the largest constraint, but, without adequate budgetary data, the magnitude of the problem is uncertain. The bulk of state revenues is derived from receipts from enterprises and institutions and levies on commerce and industrial and agricultural production. As noted in the opening pages of this chapter, both the agricultural and industrial sectors of the economy had gone into serious decline. There is virtually no way government revenues could have remained at pre-Leap levels. One former Ministry of Finance employee asserts that total government revenue declined by about 50 percent.[58] Irrespective of the precise figure, such declines echoed throughout the economy, producing budgetary and capital shortages. Given the decline in health personnel and services that all refugees and the media freely report, it is apparent that the Wei-sheng-pu came in for its share of budget cuts during this period. What degree of overspending occurred is unknown, though there are hints that deficits were incurred.

Within this generally constrained situation, however, Ministry leaders had several resources. The failure of the Leap and the reinfection of supposedly parasite-free areas,[59] as one informant said, convinced Ministry leaders that "progress needs a basis."[60] That basis had to be science. A well-known Canadian neurosurgeon, Doctor Wilder Penfield, talked to Vice-Minister of Public Health Tsui I-t'ien and other health officials in 1962. After his discussions, Penfield concluded that "There is a general expectation among them that science and higher education will solve the unresolved problems. . . ."[61]

Not only could China profitably draw upon the experiences and discoveries of her own scientists, there was an increasing willingness to tap the experiences and knowledge of the international scientific community. The number of foreign medical delegations to China reached an all-time high in 1964.[62] In addition, the Chinese Medical Association encouraged many overseas Chinese physicians to come, live, and work in China; an undetermined number did so.

The final resource which Wei-sheng-pu leaders believed they had was their ability to increase system efficiency. "Efficiency" became a much more substantial determinant of resource allocation, though certainly not the only one, as was subsequently charged. While there was an attempt to make the county hospitals serve a more extensive area, there was also the countervailing tendency to try to reduce the rate of referral to urban facilities.

Summarizing, the Ministry believed that it had several resources: (1) Doctors and other personnel were prepared to cooperate in emphasizing "standards." (2) The demise of commune clinics and the mass campaigns eliminated two competing sources of demand for drugs, equipment, and manpower. (3) The Center was actively encouraging the use of both foreign and domestic expertise. (4) The Ministry continued to believe, as it always had, that system efficiency could be improved through the application of correct management techniques. (5) Finally, those sectors of society that might have opposed these policies (e.g., Mao at the Center, cadres in the communes and Nine Man Sub-committee, and some urbanites and ruralites) were either too weakened politically, or too preoccupied with their own problems, to rate health policy a very high priority.

What is significant about these resources is that their definition and utilization was a political act. The reliance upon experts could be construed as an attempt to create a "new class." The centralization of management and economic control

144

(as happened in the pharmaceutical industry),[63] could be portrayed as an attempt to gather power in the hands of a few. The emphasis on reducing "inefficient" facilities and on denying attention to "frivolous" cases could be seen as callousness vis à vis the "masses."

While the conservation and allocation of resources were essential in the early 1960s, they had staggering political costs that only became apparent in the latter half of the decade. Once the immediate economic crisis had passed, and people began to feel that health care was a significant priority once again, those individuals responsible for retrenchment policies were vulnerable to attack from people who had been "injured" by such directives. Perhaps the greatest irony of the Cultural Revolution would be its mobilization of individuals with personal grievances to achieve the "selfless" state.

SUMMARY

The linchpin of the Great Leap strategy had been anticipated increases in agricultural and industrial production. These increases were to be generated by the massive application of labor. The expected increases were to have supported commune social welfare activities on an unparalleled scale. In turn, the provision of these services was supposed to have created a healthier and more enthusiastic peasantry; this would be reflected in still higher agricultural production. When, however, the drive was accompanied by a decline in agricultural production, the economic basis for rural welfare was gone, along with rural morale.

Important political changes occurred in each of the three policy-making arenas as a consequence of these difficulties. In the communes, wealthier brigades and relatively healthy individuals wanted to pull out from health schemes because they were subsidizing other units and individuals. In addition, the organizational and population prerequisites for a meaningful health program had been eliminated by the reduction in unit size and the concurrent devolution of economic authority within the communes. Finally, in political terms, authority was now in the hands of local leaders who were most concerned with production and least with welfare programs.

Equally important changes occurred in the Nine
Man Sub-committee. In the first instance, members
of the Sub-committee, for a complex set of reasons,
were now unwilling to support widespread mass campaigns. They so voted in late 1960. The Chairman's
support had eroded within the organization. Additionally, the Party structure below the Sub-committee had been severely weakened. Provincial and
County Party Committees were now preoccupied with
production and were unwilling to invest material and
human resources in mass campaigns which alienated
the producers they were seeking to motivate. Finally, with the communes reduced in size, and the
devolution of authority to leaders with stronger
local ties, neither the organizational nor political
foundations for mobilization existed.

In the Wei-sheng-pu, political changes were
substantial and reflected the need to make policy
congruent with the new situation; that situation
being the reduction in the number of rural health
centers, their changed financial status, the increased rate of illness, and the pressures which all
these factors generated for the urban clinical system. All the leadership changes which occurred in
the Ministry reinforced the role of medical professionals. Doctors in medical facilities played an
increasingly visible and important role in local
medical decision-making.

In conclusion, the political landscape had
changed in every major seat of policy-making. The
policy changes we shall examine in the next chapter
were not the results of a Machiavellian plot by
"capitalist roaders" as much Cultural Revolution
rhetoric suggests. Instead, those guidelines were
the reflection of differential responses among
several policy-making arenas to agricultural failure.
There was no way to insulate an agricultural economy from the consequences of agricultural disaster.

NOTES

1. Alexander Eckstein, "Economic Growth and Change
in China: A Twenty-Year Perspective," China Quarterly (hereafter CQ), no. 54 (1973), p. 216.

2. Eckstein, p. 216.

3. Eckstein, p. 216.

4. Eckstein, p. 224.

5. Eckstein, p. 229.

6. Edward Rice, Mao's Way (Berkeley: University of California Press, 1974), p. 181.

7. J. Chester Cheng, ed., The Politics of the Chinese Red Army (Stanford: Hoover Institution Publications, 1966), p. 171.

8. Chieh-fang Jih-pao [Liberation daily], August 3, 1960.

9. Ho Piao, "Wei-sheng-pu-men Ying Pa Chih-yüan Nung-yeh Tso Wei Shou-yao Jen-wu" [Health units should have the aiding of agriculture as its primary task], Hung Ch'i [Red flag], no. 18 (1960), p. 13.

10. Mao Tse-tung, "Tsai I-ts'e Hui-pao-shih Te Ch'a-hua" [Remarks at a briefing] (March 1964), in Mao Tse-tung Ssu-hsiang Wan-sui [Long live the thought of Mao Tse-tung] (Peking: 1969), p. 479.

11. Michel Oksenberg, "Occupational Groups in Chinese Society and the Cultural Revolution," The Cultural Revolution 1967 in Review, University of Michigan Papers in Chinese Studies, no. 2 (Ann Arbor: Center for Chinese Studies, 1968), p. 5.

12. Jen-min Jih-pao [People's daily], January 24, 1964.

13. Hsin Jen Wei [New people's health] (Peking: People's Health Press, 1967), pp. 11-12.

14. Mao Tse-tung, "Kuan-yü Pao-chien Kung-tso Te Chiang-hua" [Speech on health work], in Mao Tse-tung Ssu-hsiang Wan-sui, p. 454.

15. Hsin Jen Wei [New people's health], p. 13.

16. Cited in G. William Skinner, "Marketing and Social Structure in Rural China," Part 3, Journal of Asian Studies 24 (1965):397; see also, Cheng, pp. 465-529.

17. Ezra Vogel, Canton Under Communism (Cambridge: Harvard University Press, 1969), p. 282.

18. Audrey Donnithorne, China's Economic System (New York: Praeger, 1967), pp. 66-67.

19. Jen-min Shou-ts'e, 1964 [People's handbook, 1964] (Peking: Ta-kung Pao She, 1964), p. 275; see also, Donald W. Klein and Anne B. Clark, Biographic Dictionary of Chinese Communism (Cambridge: Harvard University Press, 1971), pp. 576-577.

20. Klein and Clark, p. 570.

21. Ch'üan-wu-ti [Invincible], no. 9, p. 2.

22. Klein and Clark, p. 967; see also, Union Research Service, June 19, 1970, pp. 1-11.

23. "Monstrous Crimes of Urban 'Lords' Health Ministry in Opposing June 26 Directive," Hung-i Chan-pao, Pa I Pa Chan-pao [Red medical combat bulletin and August 18 combat bulletin], June 26, 1967.

24. There are two ambiguities: First, there is little way in which one can document these attitudinal changes and there is no precise definition of professionalization, though a large literature on the subject exists. See, Peter Blau and R. W. Scott, Formal Organizations (San Francisco: Chandler, 1962); see also, Howard Vollmer and Donald Mills, Professionalism (New Jersey: Prentice-Hall, 1966), pp. 60-62.

25. Ch'üan wu-ti [Invincible], no. 16, p. 2.

26. David M. Lampton, Interview File 21 E.

27. Vogel, p. 291.

28. C. S. Chen and C. P. Ridley, Rural People's Communes in Lien-chiang (Stanford: Hoover Institution Publications, 1969); see also, Cheng.

29. Ho Ch'i, "Studies on Malaria in New China," Chinese Medical Journal 84 (1965):494-495.

30. "The Urgent Need of Improving Health in Huilai Hsien Town," Nan-fang Jih-pao [Southern daily], May 21, 1964, in Survey of the China Mainland Press (hereafter SCMP), no. 3240, p. 19.

31. "Pay Good Attention to Health Work," Nan-fang Jih-pao [Southern daily], September 28, 1960, in Current Background (hereafter CB), no. 645, pp. 16-17.

32. P'eng Teh-huai, "P'eng Teh-huai's 'Letter of Opinion'," in The Case of P'eng Teh-huai, 1959-1968 (Hong Kong: Union Research Institute, 1968), p. 11.

33. Merle Goldman, "Party Policies Toward the Intellectuals: The Unique Blooming and Contending of 1961-2," Party Leadership and Revolutionary Power in China, ed. John W. Lewis (New York: Cambridge University Press, 1970), pp. 268-303.

34. Ch'üan-wu-ti [Invincible], no. 14, p. 2.

35. Mao Tse-tung, "Tsai Pa-chieh Chiu Chung Ch'üan-hui-shang Te Chiang-hua" [Speech at the Ninth Plenum of the Eighth Central Committee] (January 18, 1961), in Mao Tse-tung Ssu-hsiang Wan-sui [Long live the thought of Mao Tse-tung] (Peking: 1967), p. 265.

36. Donnithorne, p. 74; see also, Vogel, p. 281; see also, Ezra Vogel, Interview No. 7, p. 2.

37. "An Investigation Report on How the Ch'ünhsing Brigade in Ch'üchiang Hsien, Kwangtung Province Firmly Adheres to Cooperative Medical Service Over the Past Eleven Years," Hung Ch'i [Red flag], no. 1 (1969), in Selections from China Mainland Magazines (hereafter SCMM), no. 642, pp. 27 and 31.

38. "Chieh-ho Wei-sheng Kung-tso" [Unify health work], Kuang-ming Jih-pao [Bright daily], January 16, 1961.

39. Ho Piao, p. 19.

40. "An Investigation Report on How Ch'ünhsing Brigade . . .," p. 31.

41. Cheng, p. 527.

42. David M. Lampton, Interview File 21 E, no. 4, p. 2.

43. David M. Lampton, Interview File 21 E, no. 1, p. 1.

44. Kuang-ming Jih-pao [Bright daily], June 6, 1962, in SCMP, no. 2842, pp. 14-15.

45. "T'ao Chu's Report to Higher Intellectuals," (September 28, 1961), in SCMP, no. 4200, p. 14.

46. Donnithorne, pp. 366-367.

47. "Ch'üan-kuo Yao-cheng Hui-i Tsung-chieh Ching-yan Chüeh-ting Chin-nien Fang-chen Jen-wu" [National drug conference summarizes experience and fixes the direction of this year's tasks], Kuang-ming Jih-pao [Bright daily], January 16, 1961.

48. Oksenberg, pp. 4-5.

49. China Topics, YB 584 (May 1973), p. 2.

50. Donnithorne, pp. 69-70.

51. Chu-yuan Cheng, "Health Manpower: Growth and Distribution," Public Health in the People's Republic of China, ed. Myron E. Wegman, Tsung-yi Lin, and Elizabeth F. Purcell (New York: Josiah Macy, Jr. Foundation, 1973), p. 144.

52. "The Orientation of the Revolution in Medical Education as Seen in the Growth of 'Barefoot Doctors'," Hung Ch'i [Red flag], no. 3 (1968), cited in China's Medicine 10 (1968):574-575.

53. David M. Lampton, Interview File 21 E.

54. "Mayflies Lightly Plot to Topple Giant Tree," Ch'üan-wu-ti [Invincible], June 26, 1967.

55. "T'ao Chu's Report to Higher Intellectuals," p. 15.

56. David M. Lampton, Interview File 21 E.

57. Han Kuang, "Several Problems Concerning Technical Work in Industry," Hung Ch'i [Red flag], no. 24 (1961), pp. 1-7.

58. Richard Tiao, Communist China's Finance in 1964 (Hong Kong: Union Research Institute, 1965), pp. 3-4; see also, Donnithorne, pp. 366-367.

59. "Strive to Eradicate Schistosomiasis on the Basis of Achievements Already Made," Jen-min Jih-pao [People's daily], January 24, 1964, in SCMP, no. 3160, p. 5. "Those who have been cured of this disease may be affected by it again. It is impossible to wipe out all snails within a short time . . ."

60. David M. Lampton, Interview File 21 E.

61. Wilder Penfield, "Oriental Renaissance in Education and Medicine," Science 141 (1963):1153-1161.

62. David M. Lampton, "Health Policy During the Great Leap Forward," CQ, no. 60 (1974), p. 671.

63. Ching-chi P'i-p'ing [Economic criticism] 4 (May 20, 1967).

Chapter 7
THE POLICY CONSEQUENCES OF AGRICULTURAL SETBACKS (1960-1965)

<u>INTRODUCTION</u>

In good Marxist fashion we have seen, and will continue to see, that the economy is the substructure upon which changes in the superstructure occur. Unlike Marx, however, we have seen that economic deprivation produces, at least in the short-run, conservatism rather than a revolutionary upsurge. Among leadership and nonleadership sectors of the society alike, it generates a desire to follow more traditional patterns of interaction. Economic failure necessitated alterations in the site of policy-making and produced changes in leadership composition and attitudes in each of the three policy-making arenas. These changes form the major part of the explanation for policy change in the issue areas examined below. In the course of looking at these policies, we shall begin to analyze the pressures which were impelling the system toward the Great Proletarian Cultural Revolution.

<u>ACTION POLICIES</u>

Policy retrenchment is generally less well documented than policy during periods of confidence and progress. Consequently, the analyst must often look at system performance and relate this to scraps of policy which presumably undergirded such motion.

<u>Higher medical education</u>. The most dependable figures on medical education deal with the annual number of graduates. During the Great Leap Forward, enrollment in higher-level medical schools increased rapidly, with the most dramatic increases occurring in less prestigious institutions. If it is assumed that there is about a four to five year lag between a decision to increase or decrease enrollments and this decision's reflection in the graduation figures,

Table 1 indicates that the crest of admissions to higher medical schools was reached around the 1958-1959 period (see Table 1).[1]

TABLE 1

Graduates of Higher Medical Institutions, 1956-1966

Year	Number Graduated	Percent of Total
1956-57	6,200	11.1
1957-58	5,393	7.5
1958-59	9,000	12.9
1959-60	10,500	7.8
1960-61	19,000	11.7
1961-62	17,000	9.6
1962-63	25,000	12.5
1963-64	23,000	11.5
1964-65	19,000	11.2
1965-66	19,000	11.2

Source: Chu-yuan Cheng, "Health Manpower: Growth and Distribution," in Public Health in the People's Republic of China, ed. by Myron E. Wegman, Tsung-yi Lin, and Elizabeth F. Purcell (New York: Josiah Macy, Jr. Foundation, 1973), p. 147.

By the academic year 1964-1965, the annual number of graduates from higher medical schools was, once again, at the same level as it had been prior to the expansion. The data in Table 1 indicate that the decision to reduce enrollments was made around 1960. Chu-yuan Cheng notes that by 1963, the number of medical colleges had been reduced from a 1959 high of 142 to 98.[2] What reductions in facilities did occur were most pronounced at those levels at which expansion had been most rapid during the Leap (e.g., less prestigious institutions giving intermediate medical education and provincial-level medical schools). The foundations for this policy were put into place by Vice-Minister Hsu Yun-pei in May 1960.

> . . . we must first of all strengthen the Party's leadership and then steadily increase the number of highly qualified medical workers, expand basic constructions and increase equipment and facilities, thereby enabling the county level hospitals to assume the role of

153

centers of medical technology and bases for training health cadres.[3]

Mao's attitude toward these changes is uncertain. We do know that in January 1960, Mao had proposed that higher degrees should not be emphasized; Teng Hsiao-p'ing and the Ministry of Public Health opposed this.[4] Yet, arguments over relative emphasis do not conclusively demonstrate a "line struggle." Mao's remarks at a 1964 educational conference indicate that he was in fundamental agreement with most persons (including P'eng Chen and Liu Shao-ch'i?) in calling for a "varied approach" to education, placing increased emphasis on peasant enrollments, shorter primary education, and more investment in rural education. A short dialogue reveals Mao's attitude toward medical education.

> XX [P'eng Chen?]: Except for some special cases, colleges will have three kinds of school terms: the six-year school term principally for medicine, the five-year terms for physics and engineering, and the four-year term for liberal arts. . . . In the future, school terms will be more varied in form.

> Mao: That's it, we must take a varied approach.[5]

In short, the degree to which medical education was an issue in the 1960-1964 period is debatable. It is clear that the emphasis may have been more professional than Mao would have wished, but he does not appear to have raised fundamental objections at this point. The reasons for this are rather clear. The absence of resources simply precluded most alternatives.

Contrary to much speculation about centralizing tendencies within the state structure during this period, once general policy had been formulated in Peking, local institutions had more leeway in shaping policies to meet their own needs. One manifestation of this was the increased influence of professional staff in the hospitals and medical colleges, especially in curriculum and budgetary matters. As one interviewee put it, "The system wasn't too different from the one in the United States."[6] Reflective of this input was the fact that the time devoted to political study in the medical schools declined. In 1960, Dr. Thomas Stapleton noted that 9 percent of course hours were devoted to politics;[7] by 1963, at least at China Medical College, the time had been reduced to 3.5 percent.[8]

Simultaneously, the Ministry began (1962) to gradually make all higher medical schools provide six-year courses, not just "key schools."[9] This program was never fully implemented because of financial constraints and the advent of the Cultural Revolution. In 1962, Dr. Penfield noted that "Of the other medical colleges, one-third now provide a 6-year curriculum and less than two-thirds, a 5-year curriculum. A very few schools have a 3-year course, which is intended to prepare men for the practical needs of factories, mines, and farms."[10] "In the last three years [1960-1963] they have rapidly been changing their medical schools by lengthening the curriculum and decreasing the number in each class."[11]

Elevated admissions standards accompanied lengthened curricula. Doctors who had weathered the Leap noted that heterogeneous classes had been difficult to teach. In order to rectify that situation, national medical boards were administered to applicants. One visitor observed, "The students came from all categories, but, as one would expect, the sons and daughters of well-educated parents are proportionally the most numerous."[12] One respondent explained,

> . . . actually there were few only who belonged
> to the poorer classes and . . . most of the
> students seemed to come from better class
> families . . . this was possibly due to the
> fact that poorer class families were formerly
> unable to send their children to school and
> they started school very late so that their
> background was not so good and the Medical
> School Entrance Examination [was] rather more
> difficult than [for] other courses.[13]

By 1964, the Chinese leadership was in fundamental agreement that these trends had produced an urban bias. At a major 1964 meeting on education, there was a consensus that failure to use varied teaching techniques ". . . has caused a decline in the number of students, a decline in the number of poor and lower-middle peasant students. The number of poor and lower-middle peasants without education is large."[14]

Did these policies of lengthened curricula, higher standards, and increased professional influence represent a substantial departure from the practices of the past? In the "elite" schools, retrenchment standards were only slightly more pronounced than they had been during the Leap, when

Premier Chou emphasized "key schools." In less prestigious institutions, longer curricula and reduced enrollments were more noticeable because these facilities had been most overburdened in the first place. There was a symmetry of interest between administrators and medical professionals; both wanted a reduction of burdens and a reimposition of quality. Policy reflected this symmetry.

Middle-level medical education. This is a category of training which includes physicians with intermediate-length medical education, technicians, and nurses. There was a substantial reduction in the number of such personnel being produced. This drop was at least 50 percent and, if Red Guard documents are even remotely accurate, the decline was far more enormous, with a reduction from 280,000 to 40,000 by 1964.[15]

The primary reason for this decline was that middle medical education had been the primary responsibility of provincial and county governments; they were in no financial position to support massive training programs. In addition, with reemphasis on the county hospital system, there was a reduced institutional demand for such personnel. Dr. John Bryant makes the general point that the problem with paraprofessionals is that often they are too great a burden for a rural village but incapable of doing the tasks required at the next higher stage in the referral chain.[16] Finally, because middle-level facilities had been marginal and undercapitalized, they were the most expendable when the financial squeeze came.

Lower-level medical education. This category of training encompassed a "potpourri" of health workers in communes, factories, and residential areas. The duration of their education could be measured in weeks and the county or urban district generally had been responsible for their training. The production of health workers had been part of the leviathan effort to bring some medical care to all Chinese. In 1958, there were about 2.16 million medical personnel, of which approximately 1.77 million were lower-level medical workers. By 1963, the number of lower-level personnel had declined by about 760,000;[17] this represents a decline of about 43 percent.

The case of a county near Shanghai illustrates these trends. During the Leap there had been 3,900 "health workers" in more than 2,500 production brigades. By August 1961, this number was 300.[18] There were several reasons for this decline. First,

156

making the production team the basic accounting unit
meant that each team member's income was visibly
tied to the productivity of his neighbor; people
were less willing to tolerate marginally productive
persons. In addition, "barefoot doctors" (though
not all health workers) were given work points. As
rural incomes dropped, people became less willing to
see the value of their work points diluted. The
peasant had to ask, are these people of sufficient
value that I should lose immediately needed income?
In most cases the answer appears to have been NO!
The coup de grâce to the program was the inability
of county and district facilities to adequately
train these personnel in the face of the competing
demands of patients in hospitals.

In brief, changes in all dimensions of medical
education were substantial, reflecting the diverse
pressures of different levels of the society. The
reemphasis on higher medical education reflected
the previous dissatisfactions of professionals, the
concern of those in charge of the culture and education realms, the "objective" needs of the hospital
system, and the relatively stronger financial position of higher-level institutions. Severe reductions at the middle and lower levels of the educational system reflected the weak financial and
facility position of these institutions, the lack
of demand for this type of personnel, and the severe
financial constraints in the rural areas.

Policy vis à vis medical research. The Great
Leap had not been directed against medical researchers, though it had proven difficult to insulate
them from some of the excesses of the movement.
Once the failure of the Leap had become apparent,
the line toward professionals of all types became
less ambiguous. In his already mentioned "Report
to Higher Intellectuals," T'ao Chu basically told
political zealots to leave research alone.[19] Ch'en
I made the same points in Canton.[20] This policy
persisted until 1965-1966, despite the "Socialist
Education Campaign" and the "unique blooming and
contending period" of 1961-1962, which ended in a
crackdown on certain literary personalities, especially those in Peking.

The principal guidelines for medical research
were established at the National Conference on Medical Science in March 1963. Although no copy of the
meeting's recommendations is available, we do know
that,

> More than 200 experts in western and tradition-
> al Chinese medicine and outstanding medical

scientists from various parts of the country
attended a recent National Medical Science
Conference in Peking sponsored by the Ministry
of Public Health. The meeting summed up the
achievements and experience of recent years,
set the main tasks of medical research and
worked out long-term plans for the development
of medical science.[21]

The fact that experts were so prominent at this
meeting was the basis for later Red Guard charges
(1967) that ". . . the absolute majority [of persons]
at this meeting were bourgeois specialists."[22]

Because the <u>Wei-sheng-pu</u> was the major site at
which medical research policy was being made, men
like Vice-Minister Ch'ien Hsin-chung, with their
universally acknowledged pro-research propensities,
and the Scientific Committee on Medical Sciences,
shaped policy. It was later alleged, for instance,
that Ch'ien played a crucial role at the 1963
meeting.

In 1963, the 10-Year Plan for Medical Science
was established, and originally it had only 23
research topics which were intimately related
to the people's livelihood and national defense
and construction, but Ch'ien Hsin-chung, in
order to represent the specialists, allowed the
tasks which specialists chose to enter into
the national plan, and this influenced the
completion of the major national tasks, and
[Ch'ien] allowed several bourgeois specialists
to utilize the nation's money and manpower to
achieve their . . . objectives.[23]

Concisely, the indictment was that the hapless vice-
minister permitted researchers to predominate in
the definition of scientific tasks.

The actual content of research policy reflected
the above forces, especially once the economy was on
the road to recovery. In 1963, it was announced
that,"All institutes have appointed assistants to
help experienced professors and allow ample time for
them to do research work and train young teachers
and post-graduates."[24] The subjects being investi-
gated included the transplantation of teeth, cancer,
the treatment of severe burns, and brain and open-
heart surgery. Open-heart surgery was of such high
priority that famous cardiac surgeons such as Shih
Mei-hsin were given authority to establish surgical
units. Surgeons at this level were given direct
access to vice-ministers.[25]

Research policy demonstrates how shared values
between policy-makers and professionals, and the
need to consult, shaped policy. Scientific guidelines were also affected by the fact that previous
mass campaigns (such as the drive to wipe out
schistosomiasis) had foundered because the requisite
research was absent. Finally, the elimination of
competing arenas, the decline of Mao's influence (or
interest) over research, and the accelerating economy all made the increasing impact of professionals
possible. Concluding, institutional, economic, and
power relationships were such that research thrived
during this period.

Health care delivery and the structure of the
system. Policy in this area changed substantially
because it had been most dependent on the success of
the Leap strategy itself. Vice-Minister Ho Piao
articulated the new policy in September 1960, when
he emphasized that county hospitals were to be the
hub of curative care in the countryside. To
strengthen the rural medical and health organization . . . "the county hospital must be the center. . . ."26 As we will remember, this had been
the preferred policy of the Wei-sheng-pu all along.

An entire galaxy of forces, of both rural and
urban origin, produced this policy. First, cooper-
atively financed rural centers were quite simply no
longer viable when the economic squeeze came in 1959
and 1960. As Vice-Minister of Public Health Chang
Kai observed,

> On the basis of the economic condition in the
> countryside, with the exception of a few rural
> basic-level health organizations (mainly in
> minority areas and remote border regions) which
> are established by the state and a certain
> number of health organizations which are set
> up by financially better-off communes and pro-
> duction brigades, they are, basically speaking
> and as a major means of operation, collectively
> run by medical doctors.27

As prior to the Leap, that medical care which was
available in rural areas was paid for on a fee-for-
service basis. Once the "free" aspect of commune
health care was gone, ruralites often decided that
it was preferable to take a chance on getting ill
and going to the county hospital where they would
pay if need be. Peasants made a candid assessment
of how their income could best be spent. In the
1960-1964 period, with only fee-for-service

159

traditional doctors in local group practices (united clinics), it made sense to go to the county hospital. As far as quality of service was concerned, this had been true during the Leap as well. One could cogently argue that the Ministry was actually responding to decisions made in communes, rather than formulating policy out of whole cloth. The independent decisions of millions of peasants, in the aggregate, made "free" commune health care impossible. This being the case, the Ministry had no choice but to make the county the focus of activity.

These independent decisions were reflected in the fact that by 1962 there were 70,000 rural united clinics, or about one in each of the more than 70,000 communes.[28] What happened was that old "united clinics," which had been amalgamated and taken over by communes in 1958, were disaggregated into their original component units. In most cases, these clinics were responsible for "their own profits and losses" (or fee-for-service). The Leap had succeeded in making group practice more widespread in rural areas; it failed to significantly improve the quality of personnel rendering care and was unable to make "free" medical service available on a permanent basis.

Physicians were a force behind restoring county hospitals to centrality as well. Fang Hsien-chih, in a speech to the Second Session of the Second National People's Congress, said, "Above all, we must use the hospital as the center for strengthening various phases of medical care and treatment."[29]

Wei-sheng-pu health care delivery policy reflected the concerns of other sectors of the society as well. Urbanites (especially Party cadres, insured workers, and government employees) felt that the Leap's rural emphasis had reduced their access to quality medical service. As Vice-Minister Ho Piao observed,

> Some comrades maintain arbitrarily that health work in cities is heavy already, and worry that supporting agriculture will influence urban health work.[30]

Not only was there a diffuse urban desire for better health care, these demands had powerful allies. One excellent example of this was the situation in Peking. Mayor P'eng Chen was known among doctors as a promoter of the capital, generally, and medicine specifically. In view of Peking's aging leadership and the pre-liberation concentration of services in

the capital, the relative abundance of medical
facilities in that city is not surprising. However,
P'eng was always pushing for still greater emphasis
on "his city," hoping to make it the center of brain,
thoracic, and heart surgery. As one interviewee
noted, P'eng "wanted to make Peking a beautiful
piece of crystal."[31] While we know very little
about the mechanisms by which urban interests were
articulated and advanced, looking at the concentration of resources in Shanghai and other cities, it
is apparent that other municipal leaders must have
also pushed for emphasis on their localities.[32]

In short, there was a confluence of interests
pushing for an urban-biased delivery system.
Peasants wanted to unburden themselves of economic
obligations. The Ministry needed to make the most
efficient use of its scarce monetary and manpower
resources; it argued that county hospitals were the
optimal level for health delivery. Doctors wanted
to work in the relatively structured environment of
an urban hospital. Finally, urbanites and powerful
city leaders had a stake in improvement of urban
facilities.

Political controversy did not end with the
decision to emphasize county hospitals. Upgrading
county facilities meant that major urban medical
facilities (generally at the provincial level) would
be requested to transfer personnel to these units,
on a rotating basis.[33] The response to this policy
was that major urban medical units generally sent
their least experienced physicians to county hospitals,[34] or used the threat of transfer as a means
by which to subdue truculent doctors. In addition,
when sending staff could not be avoided, they were
most often three-year doctors.[35] In short, urban
medical facilities made every attempt to hang on to
their overworked staffs; this created inequalities
and resistances between large and small cities.

Another political thicket concerned patterns of
distribution of health services within urban areas.
While a few figures on intraurban distribution of
free and insured medical services are available for
periods prior to 1959, no such data are available
covering the 1960-1965 period. As noted in earlier
chapters, no more than one-fourth of the city populace could entirely avoid directly paying for medical care. Nothing in the Leap or retrenchment
periods suggests that coverage was broadened.

. . . while the administration of labor insurance schemes . . . forms a large part of the

161

> duties of trade unions, in 1957 scarcely more
> than 70 percent of their members can have been
> covered by these schemes, while only 40 percent
> enjoyed free medical care. . . . Despite any
> subsequent extensions which may have come
> about, comprehensive coverage of the labor
> force was not approached in any year for which
> figures are available. Numbers benefiting from
> free medical care were even more restricted and
> increased much more slowly than in the case of
> labor insurance.[36]

Many urbanites were either dependents, retired persons, employees of small commercial concerns, or temporary, part-time, or contract laborers. None of these persons enjoyed free or insured medical care. While the Chinese authorities have never discussed the reasons for their failure to universalize free care, it is clear that the budgetary burdens would have been overwhelming, that fees inhibited overutilization, and that past experience indicated that when fees were removed, health costs jumped.

It seems that in circumstances of scarcity, particularly when that commodity is health care, one finds that those with political or bureaucratic power make sure that they and their families receive preferential treatment. While cadres had always received favored access to curative facilities, this became an increasingly abrasive phenomenon in the context of the early 1960s. A few excerpts from interviews will illustrate the inequities and their impact upon the public's consciousness.

> If the person was an important Party member or
> the highest class doctor or intellectual in
> another field, then he would be given the
> better quality drug whether his sickness was
> serious or not.[37]

[or]

> After 1953, she said, the Party persons wanted
> a famous doctor to take care of them and that
> inequalities in access . . . began to arise
> . . . the Great Leap Forward had not stopped
> this trend. . . . Also, she noted that heads
> of departments and above could go to Hsieh-ho
> I-yuan [Union Hospital].[38]

[or]

162

There are however in each large hospital several single rooms provided for higher-up Party
members, and these people are the only ones who
are allowed such privileges. Rank 13 upwards
may have single bed sitting rooms, furnished
with sofas and chairs and extremely comfor-
table.[39]

Even in the absence of any formal policy to
give cadres special treatment, doctors felt constrained to do so, if for no other reason than the
desire not to antagonize those who could make one's
life miserable. The distribution of health services
underscores what had become an interlocking direc-
torate of professionals, bureaucrats, and Party members. Once physicians varied treatment according
to status, disillusionment among other patients
set in.[40] This was part of the reservoir of hostility that would be mobilized in the Cultural Revolution.

Health care financing, as it related to the
communes, was defined by Vice-Minister of Public
Health Hsu Yun-pei in May 1960, and redefined by his
colleague Ho Piao in September. Hsu said,

At present, the ideal medical care system for
commune members, in view of the present level
of production and consciousness of the masses,
is collective medical care. Under this system,
the expenses for medical care are jointly
shouldered by the individual members and the
commune, and the funds are pooled and used
collectively.[41]

Hsu was, in effect, acknowledging that free medical
care was impractical and was asking ruralites to
make direct monetary contributions to health funds.
In the conditions of increasing economic scarcity
which prevailed in 1960, peasants resisted any
additional economic burdens. In September, Ho Piao
carried the retrenchment a step further by making
the plan optional.

Based on the production level of different areas
and the willingness of the masses, the payment
of a medical fee by members is by annual contribution of a health protection fee to be combined with the public welfare fund of the commune, and to be spent in a unified and even
manner.[42]

163

Not only was the ability and willingness of peasants to contribute money to the health funds decreasing, communes were becoming less and less able to make their contributions as well. Because the magnitude of welfare funds was directly tied to agricultural production, as farm output decreased so did the size of such funds. Also, the percentage of total production to be set aside for welfare purposes was reduced by governmental directive.[43]

The 1962 data for Hu Li Production Brigade (Lien-chiang County) merit a close look. Hu Li had 411 households with a total population of 1,763 persons. The brigade's welfare fund was 2,986¥, or about 1.6¥ per capita.[44] Expenses for entertainment, relief, health care, and supplementary grain rations all were paid from this fund. Consequently, only a small portion of that 1.6¥ was available for health care. If Hu Li was even in the approximate position of the already mentioned Ch'unhsing Brigade, more people were getting sick. If 2 percent of Hu Li's population was "seriously ill" (and each required an outlay of even 100¥), the welfare fund would have been more than exhausted by emergency health demands alone.

In the face of these economic constraints, commune cadres had only three choices: get commune members to pick up the financial slack, obtain central subsidy, or let each family shift for itself. Because peasant incomes were linked to production in the same direct way as were commune welfare funds, increasing the levies on commune members offered no solution. In addition, in the face of material scarcities, marginal commune health facilities had decreasing relative utility. One brigade member said, "Those who are sick should pay for themselves."[45]

Trying to obtain central subsidies proved just as difficult because state revenues were ultimately tied to the agricultural base also. We have found no instance in which the central budget was able to bail out floundering commune health centers, at this time, with the exception of a few in strategic border areas populated by minority peoples. Consequently, commune cadres would often permit locals to go to county facilities, receive care, and then not make sure that the county was reimbursed for the services rendered. As noted, this method of obtaining indirect subsidies caused county health budgets endless problems.[46] In response, hospital administrators compelled communes to sign contracts guaranteeing to pay for services received. "The

164

timing, method, and steps of the carrying out of such responsibilities have been made concrete and certain by the signing of aid contracts."[47] As a result of all these economic, administrative, and political constraints, some cadres are quoted as believing the cooperative medical service was "looking for trouble."[48] By 1964, Vice-Minister Chang Kai could confidently assert that health organizations "are, basically speaking and as a major means of operation, collectively run by medical doctors."[49]

Because change in financial policy in urban areas had been almost imperceptible during the Leap, minimal retrenchment was necessary, though the massive transfer of urbanites and cadres out of cities must have eased hospital burdens somewhat. Payment arrangements and levels of benefits appear to have remained the same, although, in the absence of budgetary figures, a full explanation for this stability is difficult to advance. One probable reason for the stability in level of benefits, despite the general economic decline, is that the heavy industrial workers entitled to insured health care drew upon a relatively stable resource base-- labor insurance funds.[50] The only other sectors of the populace entitled to free health care were Party cadres and government workers (and some students), groups which presumably had too much leverage in the system to be denied benefits.

Because the same groups remained entitled to the same level of benefits, it is not surprising that the urban hospital administrator's problems remained much the same as they had been during the previous decade; waste and "frivolous" use were public enemies number one and two.

> People will go to a doctor when they are a little indisposed, but do not make proper use of the medicine received. They do so because they think they do not have to pay. Both patients and doctors thought in these terms: ". . . the state will pay. . . ."[51]

Waste occurred not only because there was a lack of incentive for efficiency, but also because physicians and administrators felt that the prerequisite to better treatment was better equipment. The Ministry set up rigid clearing procedures for purchasing equipment and exhorted everyone to ". . . conquer the desire for the big, the new, and the foreign."

While Lardy's study of fiscal management during the 1950s makes it clear that the Great Leap did not eliminate the central government's capacity to redistribute resources,[52] once the movement ended, Peking may have reacquired more control over local expenditures through local branches of the People's Bank. In 1960 it was announced, "The expenses of the hospitals have recently been covered by the state's budget, the medical service has improved, and the various localities have further cut the medical charges."[53] Along with the increasingly active role of the Ministry in local financing, one would expect that added control over local expenditures was exerted, though we cannot be certain. A preliminary hypothesis is that retrenchment increased the percentage of locally spent revenues over which Peking had control. While this probably did not affect regional patterns of distribution, this may well have increased central leverage over expenditures.

The pharmaceutical industry was importantly affected by financial considerations and policy. Leap attempts to reduce drug prices, and thereby lighten the burdens on both the Wei-sheng-pu, commune clinics, and patients, had precipitated drastic declines in pharmaceutical quality and reliability. The ultimate solution to the "quality-quantity-price" dilemma was to reorganize the pharmaceutical industry, increase quality control, and expand the industry's productive capacity. In order to do this, a national pharmaceutical "trust," ultimately under the control of Po I-po (vice-chairman of the State Planning Commission) and the Industrial and Communications Committee (Kung Chiao Tang-wei), was established.[54] The purpose of the trust was to bring all pharmaceutical producers under unified control in order to increase supervision, provide central marketing facilities and more efficient procurement, and deny substandard producers scarce resources. By the start of the Cultural Revolution, 100 of China's 283 pharmaceutical plants were in this trust.[55] According to one interviewee, local political and economic resistances made the incorporation of all producers into the trust difficult.[56] While one would like a great deal more information about the precise calculations leading to the creation of the pharmaceutical trust, it is clear that attempts to raise drug quality and increase quantity were related to consumer dissatisfaction, the loss of confidence among doctors and pharmacists, and the need to use scarce resources efficiently.

166

Policy regarding the conditions of physician employment changed substantially. Party political "interference" in medical affairs was reduced, doctors were given a larger voice in local decision-making, and professional stratification became increasingly evident.

The enduring dilemma which the Party faced was how to "give full scope to the ability of the experts but at the same time shatter all vestiges of monopoly . . . by them." During the Leap, many zealous cadres had emphasized the latter half of the contradiction, often attempting to exercise supervision in clinical situations. The result, from both the doctor's and patient's perspective, had been a reduction in quality of care. In late 1960, Liberation Daily asserted that most scientists had been ideologically healed, the implication being that they could now be left alone. The following year, Ch'en I asserted the same thing and T'ao Chu said, Party leaders ". . . should show concern for the higher intellectuals, respect them and unite with them."[57]

This pattern of insulating professionals (and especially doctors) from political pressures persisted, despite the 1963 attacks on literary intellectuals. In 1964, the Chinese Medical Journal noted,

> These achievements are mainly due to the fact that our medical and scientific workers throughout the country have rallied around the Party and Chairman Mao and have carried out the policy of "letting a hundred flowers blossom and a hundred schools of thought contend" and of academic democracy.[58]

One of the problems that emerged during the Leap had been that exceedingly zealous cadres, in their attempts to overcome professional dominance, had denied there was any distinction to be made between doctors, nurses, and technicians. The result had been a perceived deterioration in medical service. Patients were dissatisfied and doctors were horrified by the specter of "unqualified" persons providing treatment.[59] This picture emerges from the Chinese media as well as refugees. One ward which reemphasized professional control in 1962 claimed to have realized the following gains from that move.

> Since the beginning of this year, this ward has firmly gripped strengthening the system of

technical responsibilities for doctors and
nurses and exerted its effort to carry out the
regulations and systems regarding doctors and
nurses, with the result that the rate of cure
has steadily risen, the mistakes committed by
doctors and nurses have conspicuously decreased,
the sanitation and orderliness of the ward have
also notably improved. In strengthening the
system of technical responsibilities, the No. 8
Ward pays particular attention to bringing out
the role and special qualifications of the
experienced doctors and nurses. According to
their qualifications and work requirements, the
responsibility and duty of each doctor and
nurse has been defined and the relationship of
technical guidance between the upper-level
doctors and the lower-level doctors has also
been fixed.[60]

As far as local hospital and medical school
policy-making was concerned, doctors were recruited
into "Control Committees," generally composed of one
director, or dean, and four vice-directors (each of
which was a member of the faculty). According to
Penfield, the dean was nominated by the Ministry of
Health and the Ministry of Education, but was finally appointed by the State Council. The one knowledgeable interviewee on this point observed that
these committees encouraged professionals to take
an active part in administration during the
period.

She said that at these meetings interchange was
fairly open and professionals were listened to
in making decisions. . . . She said this practice of consulting doctors about the budget
was eliminated by the end of 1965.[61]

A trend of the most momentous future importance
was the reappearance of Party recruitment policies
similar to those of 1956. Medical professionals
were brought into the Party in large (but unknown)
numbers. Marie Sieh noted in 1964, "In earlier
years only about 30 percent of the medical students
were Party or Youth League members but membership
has now risen to about 50 percent in each medical
college. Whether the student is or is not a Party
or League member may be crucial in his chances of
future research or promotion."[62] Interviews reveal
the same phenomenon. One respondent summed up the
situation by saying, "Therefore any doctor who is

really keen to get ahead and interested in his work, will either try to join the League or Party, or will attempt to leave the country."[63] Not only did opportunities for research depend on political status, so did one's capacity to avoid being sent to the countryside.

While one needed Party membership to advance professionally, this was not sufficient; one had to possess skill as well.

> If one did join the Party, respondent felt that his chances of promotion would certainly be increased, but the whole question of promotion was rather complex . . . no matter how progressive a person was, without good skill, his chances of promotion in the medical field would be almost nil.[64]

Not only was skill valued, but specific institutions had de facto recognition as most capable of producing skilled individuals. One informant noted that her medical college had never considered putting someone on the staff unless he or she had graduated from China Medical College, Peking Medical College, Shanghai First, or Chung Shan (Sun Yat-sen).[65] Students who graduated from prestigious medical schools were in an assignment category called "assignment to the whole nation."[66] Students from these institutions were generally only sent to "grade number one" cities (usually large urban areas). By the mid-1960s, then, the Party had become the main vehicle for career and geographic mobility; skill became a major criterion for Party membership. As such values and objectives increasingly permeated the organization, the homogeneity of political values eroded; the same potential for intraorganizational conflict existed in 1965-1966 as had existed in 1956-1957, with the Party split between political and more professionally oriented members.

Because the Leap had generated exceptionally heavy burdens for doctors and clinical staffs, one of the first tasks was to reduce those loads so that patients who were seen received more attention and doctors had additional time. In the process, fewer patients could be treated.

> . . . in previous years the number of patients per session had not been limited, as many as wished to register being accepted, the only limit being the time the registration office

closed, so that doctors would never know how
many patients to expect per session and the
number was generally very large, which resulted
in doctors being very overworked. . . . Around
1961 therefore this system was changed; only a
certain number being allowed to register each
day regardless of the hour of registration. . . .[67]

This problem of doctor loads and patient care brings
a dilemma facing the Ministry into sharp focus.
When doctors are overworked, patients receive poorer
care; this leads Party cadres, workers, and doctors
to demand that the medical system more adequately
meet their needs. However, if doctors reduce the
number of people seen, then those who have to wait
longer or who are not seen at all claim that the
system is not "serving the broad masses."
The final area of policy affecting the conditions of physician employment concerned the vitality
of professional life as measured by the number of
medical delegations to and from China, the number of
medical conferences held in the People's Republic,
and the number and content of medical journals
published. Between 1963 and 1965, the annual number
of medical conferences reached record levels, as did
the number of delegations to and from China.[68]
Similarly, the Chinese Medical Association noted
that ". . . the Association's journals have improved
both in quality and in quantity."[69] Finally, as the
first half of the 1960s progressed, the Chinese
Medical Journal was increasingly devoted to "pure"
research articles.[70]
There are several reasons for this increase in
professional vitality: First, economic recovery
meant that the financial underpinnings for such
activities once again existed. Secondly, several
vice-ministers of public health (e.g., Ch'ien Hsin-
chung, Fu Lien-chang, and Ho Piao) were committed
to improvements in professional life. As Ch'ien's
power within the Wei-sheng-pu increased, policies
with which he was presumably more sympathetic became
increasingly apparent, especially the importance
attached to research. Also, once the line had
become one of giving full play to scientific expertise, conferences and journals were the logical
vehicles for attaining this goal. Finally, once
the decision to play an active role in the world
scientific community had been made, China's leaders
felt constrained to meet the expectations of
foreign experts; this meant an emphasis on quality.

Policy vis à vis traditional medicine was not formally changed, although important alterations occurred in the process of implementation. The appointment of Kuo Tzu-hua as head of the Bureau of Traditional Medicine (Chung-i-ssu) was important for several reasons.[71] First, Kuo was a specialist in Chung-i and he shared the feeling of a number of respected traditional physicians that the popularization of traditional medicine tended to degrade it; if nothing else, such popularization constituted an immediate economic threat to its practitioners. Kuo and his colleagues generally opposed the "leftism which asserted that anyone can be a traditional doctor." There was a confluence of interest between western and Chinese-style physicians. Doctors of neither school wanted western-style physicians to study Chung-i.

As a consequence of this shared orientation, policy toward Chung-i gravitated toward a configuration that would antagonize the fewest persons and expend minimal resources. Research provided this common ground. As a later attack noted,

> Ever since counter-revolutionary revisionist Kuo Tzu-hua took charge of the department, he has placed the whole weight on nine research bases in the country. . . . By offering high rank and handsome emolument, he enlisted a number of "famous old herbalists" to tender their special service to a minority of people. . . . These were the very people who looked down on the herbalist teams dispatched to rural villages and doing greatly useful work there and who called them disrespectful names like "charlatans," "pumpkins," [and] "dim wits."[72]

Research had become a strategy for giving Chung-i attention without pushing programs which would be opposed by both medical communities.

While attempts had been made during the Leap to bring traditional doctors into every facet of western-style medical practice, such attempts were significantly reduced throughout the first half of the decade of the 1960s. Robert Worth relates an anecdote about the sudden shift in policy.

> In the spring of 1962 at a regular staff meeting in the hospital the Party Secretary read Chou En-lai's famous "it is more important to be expert than to be red" speech, and instantly every western-style doctor knew that

from that day on he was free to reject the
advice of the traditional practitioner if he
wished to do so.[73]

One interviewee even put it more bluntly. ". . . in
the hospital traditional doctors kept in their place
because they never were anybody anyway. . . ."[74]
     The final factor which altered the position of
traditional doctors was the decreased availability
of traditional pharmaceuticals. With agricultural
production declining rapidly, land previously
devoted to growing medicinal herbs was converted to
food production. This precipitated an increase in
the price of traditional medical preparations and
caused shortages;[75] both phenomena adversely affected
the livelihoods of traditional practitioners. The
decline in the availability of traditional pharmaceuticals, and the attendant difficulties this
created for traditional doctors, reflected less any
conscious policy of medical policy-makers than the
independent decisions of thousands of production
teams and brigades. Once again, one sees that much
health policy is made well outside of Peking. The
capacity of leaders to influence these decisions is
often marginal, at best.
     Policy vis à vis mass campaigns changed as much
as guidelines on health care delivery. This reflected the dramatic changes that had occurred within
both the Nine Man Sub-committee and the communes.
Vice-Minister Ho Piao set out the new policy in
September 1960.

          Prevention and cure of all kinds of epidemics,
          diseases from parasites and local diseases
          should be carried out as soon as the opportun-
          ity presents itself. . . .[76]

For Ho, there appeared to be no urgency in rekindling
such campaigns. Cultural Revolution charges assert
that there was a virtual alliance against more mass
health movements consisting of people at the Party
Center, professionals in the Ministry, the medical
community, and the peasants.

          The handful of capitalist roaders in the Party,
          hand in glove with the reactionary "authori-
          ties," did all they could to oppose Chairman
          Mao and block his voice. They said that the
          commune members could not understand the
          meaning of Chairman Mao's poems and that the
          mass movement was "wanton mischief."[77]

172

Not only was the morale of peasants insufficiently high to support such campaigns, the reduction in commune size (and the devolution of financial and planning authority within these smaller units) meant that the organizational basis for mass campaigns did not exist. Additionally, the Nine Man Sub-committee had voted to discontinue the campaigns in the face of the paramount need to increase agricultural production. The Ministry's feeling about mass campaigns was brutally summed up by Ch'ien Hsin-chung: "Health movement of the masses, due to lack of scientific knowledge, is as good as formalism. . . . When the dust of the earth is fanned up, that gives people more chances of inhaling viruses and spreads tuberculosis."[78]

Once the economy had picked up, Mao began to push for mass campaigns again. In January 1964, the Sub-committee met in Shanghai where it rejected proposals for renewing the movements. People's Daily summarized the meeting's findings by saying, "Schistosomiasis affects wide areas, and the factors for its outbreak are very complicated. Those who have been cured of this disease may be affected by it again. It is impossible to wipe out all snails within a short time. . . ."[79]

The result of this widespread unwillingness to launch large-scale mass campaigns was that Mao looked elsewhere in the polity for supporters. Soon after the January meeting, the People's Liberation Army emerged as the major institutional force behind mass health campaigns.

> Organs under the direct jurisdiction of the PLA Air Force are model patriotic sanitation units of the PLA and are also the red banners of the patriotic sanitation campaign in Peking and in the national patriotic sanitation campaign.[80]

Once again, one of Mao's political tactics is evident; when confronted with resistance or lethargy in one policy-making body, he sought to find another which would be a vessel of his will. The trouble was that his backers frequently defected, were coopted, or tried to acquire power themselves.

While Mao pushed for mobilization, the Wei-sheng-pu emphasized preventive tasks in industry and the cities. In each program, research was proclaimed to be the indispensable basis. This reflected the desires of Ministry experts, the medical community, and the lessons which the failures of the Leap had taught.

SUMMARY

Economic difficulties produced a reduction in
the number of policy-making arenas. The "divided"
policy-making apparatus of the Great Leap Forward
gave way to a configuration in which the Ministry
of Public Health was the major policy-making site.
The Ministry was an institution in which medical
doctors predominated. It is important to recognize,
however, that the Wei-sheng-pu did not cause the
collapse of the commune health arena or the Nine
Man Sub-committee. On the contrary, it merely
responded to their "demise" in a way that was most
congruent with its own resources, the perceptions
of its leaders, and the pressures to which it was
subjected by disenchanted sectors of the society.
Almost all political and economic factors were
pushing for policies which gave the medical system
a pronounced urban and professional bias. Peasants
could not afford commune health care and preferred
to take their chances on having to go to a county
hospital. To rural cadres, central leaders, and
members of the Nine Man Sub-committee, increased
agricultural production was the major need. Consequently, disruptive campaigns were terminated and
communes restructured in such a way as to maximize
the incentives for production. The form of organization most conducive to increasing production was
not optimal for the delivery of health care or the
promotion of mass campaigns. The Ministry believed
that health care could most efficiently be delivered
with the county hospital as the hub of activity.
The leaders of major urban centers, like Peking's
Mayor P'eng Chen, decried the deterioration in urban
health standards which the Leap had precipitated.
They argued for emphasis on their cities. In short,
most identifiable sectors of Chinese society had at
least a short-run interest in emphasizing urban
facilities and "quality" care.
While this policy initially had the support,
or at least acquiescence, of most sectors of the
polity, once economic conditions improved and
people's aspirations grew, the fact that some sectors of the population were treated "more equally"
than others produced increasing levels of hostility.
Retrenchment policies had retarded the rate of extension of health insurance, had cut the number of
students in medical schools, had reduced the rate
of expansion of health facilities, and had dashed
peasant hopes for readily available curative health
care. All of this created a reservoir of discontent

174

which could be mobilized. Mao's major political task in the second half of the 1960s was to find and mobilize these sectors of the polity in order to overcome his political opponents. This is the story to which we now turn.

NOTES

1. Accelerated graduation in the 1962-1964 period may have produced some of the bulge in the figures for these years.

2. Chu-yuan Cheng, "Health Manpower: Growth and Distribution," in Public Health in the People's Republic of China, eds. Myron Wegman, Tsung-yi Lin, and Elizabeth Purcell (New York: Josiah Macy, Jr. Foundation, 1973), pp. 146-147.

3. Hsu Yun-pei, "Advance the Great Work of Protecting the People's Health," Chinese Medical Journal 80 (1960):413.

4. Ch'üan-wu-ti [Invincible], no. 14, p. 2.

5. Mao Tse-tung, "Ch'un-chieh T'an-hua Chi-yao" [Minutes of a spring festival chat] (February 13, 1964), Mao Tse-tung Ssu-hsiang Wan-sui [Long live the thought of Mao Tse-tung] (Peking: 1969), pp. 463-464.

6. David M. Lampton, Interview File 21 E. This individual was trained in the United States.

7. Ezra Vogel, Interview No. 31, p. 3.

8. "Thoroughly Criticize and Repudiate the Eight-Year Medical Education Program Pushed by China's Krushchev," China's Medicine 3 (1968):165.

9. "Thoroughly Criticize and Repudiate . . .," p. 168.

10. Wilder Penfield, "Oriental Renaissance in Education and Medicine," Science 141 (1963):1153-1161.

11. Wilder Penfield, "Yale Reports Number 280: Interview with Dr. Wilder Penfield," China 1963: Food, Medicine, People's Communes, in Far East Reporter (n.d.), p. 25.

175

12. Penfield, "Oriental Renaissance . . .," pp.
1153-1161. Penfield notes that only one in thirty
applicants was accepted.

13. Ezra Vogel, Interview No. 22, p. 3.

14. Mao Tse-tung, "Ch'un-chieh T'an-hua Chi-yao,"
pp. 461-462.

15. "Chairman Mao's June 26 Directive," Hung-i
Chan-pao and Pa I Pa Chan-pao [Red medical combat
bulletin and August 18 combat bulletin] (June 26,
1967), in Survey of the China Mainland Press-Supplement (hereafter SCMP-S), no. 198, p. 34.

16. John Bryant, Health Care and the Developing
World (Ithaca: Cornell University Press, 1969),
p. 178.

17. The data from which these figures were gener-
ated may be found in Chu-yuan Cheng, pp. 144-145.
For the method of computation see, David M. Lampton,
"The Politics of Public Health in China: 1949-1969"
(Ph.D. diss., Stanford University, 1973), pp. 253-
254.

18. "The Orientation of the Revolution in Medical
Education as Seen in the Growth of 'Barefoot Doctors'," Hung Ch'i [Red flag], no. 3 (1968), cited
in China's Medicine 10 (1968):574-575.

19. "T'ao Chu's Report to Higher Intellectuals"
(September 28, 1961), in Survey of the China Mainland Press (hereafter SCMP), no. 4200, p. 14.

20. David M. Lampton, Interview File 21 E.

21. "National Conference on Medical Science in
Peking," New China News Agency (hereafter NCNA),
March 16, 1963, in SCMP, no. 2942, pp. 13-14.

22. Ch'üan-wu-ti [Invincible], no. 14, p. 2.

23. Ch'üan-wu-ti [Invincible], no. 14, p. 2.

24. "New China's Higher Medical Education," NCNA,
August 17, 1963, SCMP, no. 3044, p. 15.

25. David M. Lampton, Interview Files 21 E and 21 F.

26. Ho Piao, "Wei-sheng-pu-men Ying Pa Chih-yüan
Nung-yeh Tso Wei Shou-yao Jen-wu" [Health units

should have the aiding of agriculture as the primary task], Hung Ch'i [Red flag], no. 18 (1960), p. 17.

27.   Chang Kai, "Health Work Makes Big Strides in the Service of Industrial and Agricultural Production," Kuang-ming Jih-pao [Bright daily], October 6, 1964, in SCMP, no. 3339, p. 13.

28.   "Chairman Mao's June 26 Directive," p. 34.

29.   Fang Hsien-chih, "Medical Workers Must Go Out of the Hospitals to Eliminate Sickness," Joint Publications Research Service 18, no. 6623 (January 20, 1961):34.

30.   Ho Piao, p. 15.

31.   David M. Lampton, Interview File 21 E.

32.   David M. Lampton, Health, Conflict, and the Chinese Political System, Michigan Papers in Chinese Studies, no. 18 (Ann Arbor: Center for Chinese Studies, 1974), Chapter 1.

33.   Ho Piao, p. 15.

34.   "China's Hospital and Health Network," NCNA, September 27, 1964, in SCMP, no. 3309, p. 17.

35.   Ezra Vogel, Interview No. 22, p. 2.

36.   Audrey Donnithorne, China's Economic System (New York: Praeger, 1967), p. 213.

37.   Ezra Vogel, Interview No. 35, p. 7.

38.   David M. Lampton, Interview File 21 C.

39.   Ezra Vogel, Interview No. 25, p. 6.

40.   David M. Lampton, Interview File 21 E.

41.   Hsu Yun-pei, pp. 412-413.

42.   Ho Piao, p. 18.

43.   Chin Ming, "The Way in Which Financial Work in the People's Communes Serves Distribution," Hung Ch'i [Red flag], no. 22 (1960), p. 38.

44.   C. S. Chen and C. P. Ridley, Rural People's

Communes in Lien-chiang (Stanford: Hoover Institution Publications, 1969), pp. 13 and 30.

45. "An Investigation Report on How the Ch'ünhsing Brigade in Ch'üchiang Hsien, Kwangtung Province Firmly Adheres to Cooperative Medical Service Over the Past Eleven Years, Hung Ch'i [Red flag], no. 1 (1969), in Survey of China Mainland Magazines (hereafter SCMM), no. 642, p. 30.

46. Ezra Vogel, Interview No. 30, p. 5.

47. Ho Piao.

48. "An Investigation Report on How the Ch'ünhsing Brigade . . .," p. 32.

49. Chang Kai, p. 13.

50. What information is available on the size of these funds comes from the early 1950s. See Current Background (hereafter CB), no. 382, p. 21.

51. Wen-hui Pao, November 25, 1964.

52. Nicholas R. Lardy, "Centralization and Decentralization in China's Fiscal Management," China Quarterly (hereafter CQ), no. 61 (1975), pp. 25-60.

53. "Medical Fees Lowered in Various Hsien and Municipalities in Kwangtung Province," Nan-fang Jih-pao [Southern daily], August 6, 1960, SCMP, no. 2329, p. 33.

54. Ching-chi P'i-p'ing [Economic criticism] 4 (May 20, 1967).

55. "Survey Report on Conditions in Tientsin People's Pharmaceutical Plant Since Trial Operation of Trust," Ch'iu Liu Chan-pao [The root out Liu combat bulletin], June 21, 1967, in SCMP-S, no. 210, p. 23.

56. David M. Lampton, Interview with former cadre, Hong Kong, 1973.

57. "T'ao Chu's Report to Higher Intellectuals," p. 15.

58. "News and Notes," Chinese Medical Journal 83 (1964):697.

59.   David M. Lampton, Interview File 21 E.

60.   "To Fix Responsibilities and Duties of Doctors and Nurses; to Perfect Regulations and Systems," Kuang-ming Jih-pao [Bright daily], June 6, 1962, in SCMP, no. 2842, pp. 14-15; see also, pp. 16-19.

61.   David M. Lampton, Interview File 21 E.

62.   Marie Sieh, "Medicine in China: Wealth for the State," Current Scene 3, no. 5 (1964):7.

63.   Ezra Vogel, Interview No. 41, p. 1.

64.   Ezra Vogel, Interview No. 16, p. 5.

65.   David M. Lampton, Interview File 21 E.

66.   "The Medical Educational Institution in China," Interview File 21 J, p. 9.

67.   Ezra Vogel, Interview No. 37, p. 7.

68.   David M. Lampton, "Health Policy During the Great Leap Forward," CQ, no. 60 (1974), p. 671.

69.   "News and Notes," Chinese Medical Journal 83 (1964):549.

70.   David M. Lampton, "The Politics of Public Health in China: 1949-1969," pp. 251-253.

71.   "Chairman Mao's June 26 Directive," p. 32.

72.   "Chairman Mao's June 26 Directive," pp. 32-33.

73.   Robert Worth, "Institution Building in the People's Republic of China: The Rural Health Centre," unpublished manuscript, p. 13.

74.   David M. Lampton, Interview File 21 E.

75.   Ralph Croizier, Traditional Medicine in Modern China (Cambridge: Harvard University Press, 1968), p. 193; see also, "Fa-tung Ch'ün-chung Chin-chua Yao-ts'ai Sheng-ch'an" [Mobilize the masses and strengthen drug production], Kuang-ming Jih-pao [Bright daily], January 16, 1961.

76.   Ho Piao, p. 15.

77.   "Struggle Against Schistosomiasis," China's Medicine 11 (1968):672.

78.   "Chairman Mao's June 26 Directive," p.32.

79.   Jen-min Jih-pao [People's daily], January 24, 1964.

80.   Jen-min Jih-pao [People's daily], March 6, 1964, SCMP, no. 3187, p. 1.

PART 4

THE CULTURAL REVOLUTION: COALITION POLITICS

Chapter 8
MAO AND THE MINISTRY DEFINE
THE PROBLEMS: THE ORIGINS
OF THE CULTURAL REVOLUTION
IN HEALTH (JUNE 1965-AUGUST 1966)

INTRODUCTION

The political fissures which cleaved Chinese
society in the mid-1960s were so deep that they must
be specified prior to an analysis of the health
issue itself. Because medical policy is importantly
affected by debates about science, intellectuals,
social equity, and urban-rural relations, when
these issues became the focus of political controversy in the mid-1960s there was no way in which the
health system could remain insulated.

The issues which divide a political system's
leaders may be quite different from those which have
the greatest salience to the citizenry. As well,
both the political elite and the broad masses may,
themselves, be divided over various diagnoses of the
situation. For China's political elite, the central
debates of the 1965-1966 period concerned: How
accessible should the Communist Party be to external
criticism? How responsive should the Party and
government bureaucracies be to Chairman Mao's policy
initiatives? To what extent should urban-rural
equity be sacrificed in order to achieve accelerated
economic growth? Need equity be sacrificed in order
to achieve rapid growth? To what degree should the
cultural and educational systems primarily be
devoted to the task of reshaping man's nature,
creating a "new Maoist man"? What would such a man
look like? To what extent is economic development
and material plenty a precondition for ideological
change? Finally, what role should the military play
in society, how technologically sophisticated need
the armed forces be, and what political values
should such forces embody? The mid-1960s, then, was
a period during which China's leadership split over
the question of what specific intermediate-range
policies would promote the shared goals of making

China a rich, powerful, and communist country. The intensity of the debate became such that leaders began to openly question each other's devotion to the long-range objectives themselves.

The issues of importance to the Chinese populace in the mid-1960s were less abstract. Every set of developmental policies involves distributing social gains and burdens to citizens. During the retrenchment, the burdens had fallen with particular force upon identifiable sectors of the population; the favored sectors were equally conspicuous. Temporary, part-time, and contract laborers who were denied regular status in urban industries called for higher wages and additional benefits. Students who had been sent to the countryside in the late 1950s and early 1960s in order to lighten the burdens of schools and cities demanded that the regime meet their desires for urban status and career advancement. Suburban peasants who saw the relative prosperity and accouterments of urban life called for more equity. Non-Party citizens decried the injustice of cadres receiving benefits far in excess of those available to most people. In short, scarcity compelled the regime to allocate benefits; the disadvantaged sectors of the population challenged the legitimacy of such patterns of distribution.

What makes the Cultural Revolution such a unique, complex, and important period is that as the leadership fragmented, each elite splinter group sought to mobilize those segments of the society with which it shared the greatest overlap of interest. These vertical ties produced complex elite-mass coalitions, expanding political turmoil, and significant violence. It is in this context that health issues must be viewed.

The picture to emerge of Mao in the two previous chapters is that of a leader who had been unable to realize several policy objectives, a man who had focused almost exclusively on issues unrelated to health, and a man who had begun to search for new institutional allies. Only by late 1964 and 1965 did Mao take a renewed public interest in health issues. As he did, the Chairman began to specify the problems he saw.[1] In response, the Ministry of Public Health defined the situation as "it" perceived it. By August 1966, these two perceptual worlds were so divergent that Chairman Mao redefined the major issue as that of power. As in 1955 and 1956, leadership alteration had become a precondition for policy change.

Mao advertised his basic objections to previous trends in health policy in a June 1965 blast against the Wei-sheng-pu. It is a statement worth quoting at length.

Tell the Ministry of Public Health that it only works for fifteen per cent of the total population of the country and that this fifteen per cent is mainly composed of gentlemen, while the broad masses of the peasants do not get any medical treatment. First they don't have any doctors; second they don't have any medicine. The Ministry of Public Health is not a Ministry of Public Health for the people, so why not change its name to the Ministry of Urban Health, the Ministry of Gentlemen's Health, or even to Ministry of Urban Gentlemen's Health?

Medical education should be reformed. There's no need to read so many books: In medical education there is no need to accept only higher middle school graduates or lower middle school graduates. It will be enough to give three years to graduates from higher primary schools. They would then study and raise their standards mainly through practice. If this kind of doctor is sent down to the countryside, even if they haven't much talent, they would be better than quacks and witch doctors and the villages would be better able to afford to keep them. The more books one reads the more stupid one gets. . . .

They work divorced from the masses, using a great deal of manpower and materials in the study of rare, profound and difficult diseases at the so-called pinnacle of science, yet they either ignore or make little effort to study how to prevent and improve the treatment of commonly seen, frequently occurring and widespread diseases. I am not saying that we should ignore the advanced problems, but only a small quantity of manpower and material should be expended on them, while a great deal of manpower and material should be spent on the problems to which the masses most need solutions. . . .

We should leave behind in the city a few of the less able doctors who graduated one or two years ago, and the others should all go into the countryside. The "four clean-ups" movement

185

was wound up in the year xx and has been basically completed but even though the "four
clean-ups" has been completed, medical and
health work in the villages has not yet been
completed!
  In medical and health work put the emphasis
on the countryside![2]

In this pre-Cultural Revolution phase, the Chairman
articulated only general policy proposals, leaving
it to the bureaucracy to develop specific programs.
This tactic left him free to condemn future policy,
as he wished. The Wei-sheng-pu tried to keep the
level of attack from escalating by meeting some of
these demands, within the constraints that it faced.
  Regarding medical education, Mao generally
believed that it was too long and produced physicians who had a dysfunctional dependency upon technologically advanced urban hospitals. The Chairman
emphasized that "quality" medical education had produced an anti "worker-peasant" recruitment bias, a
fact with which his later opponents agreed.[3]

  Of the new students enrolled in Peking between
  1959 and 1962, only 5 percent came from worker
  or peasant families, while 30 percent came from
  families of top intellectuals.[4]

For those students with less background who had
been admitted to medical schools in the 1958-1962
period, there was a high rate of failure.[5] What Mao
professed to see, and this provided a good basis
for mobilization, was a Ministry of Health dominated
by elite doctors, trained in elite schools, selecting
elite students, to run China's urban-based hospital
system. From this perspective, medical education
was socializing the "wrong" people with the "wrong"
values.
  Mao's views on research were, at best, ambiguous
and, at worst, conceptually weak. He was concerned
that excessive attention was devoted to the "pinnacles," yet said he was not opposed to advanced
research per se. Implicit in the Chairman's view
was the assumption that sophisticated research was
less relevant to the needs of the "average" Chinese
than other possible areas of endeavor. In fact,
however, the Chinese have high rates of cancer,
cardio-vascular disease, and severe burns. In order
to solve these problems, investments in the most
sophisticated basic research were (and are) needed.
In short, Mao's uneasiness was not easily translated

186

into workable criteria for a research program. Even
two months after his June 26th directive he waffled
when talking to Ch'ien Hsin-chung and Chang Kai. He
said, "Yes, theory has to be integrated with reality!
Advanced sciences must be developed still."[6]

Mao was also distressed to note that Party
members and organs charged with overseeing medical
research had been professionalized. The State Scientific and Technological Commission, the Ministry's
Scientific Committee on Medical Sciences, and ad hoc
research policy-making bodies (e.g., the body that
formulated the Ten-Year Plan for Medical Research)
all were dominated by professionals, or were highly
responsive to them.[7] Later assertions claim that
these individuals shaped policy to reflect the needs
and desires of professionals. The already mentioned
Ten-Year Plan for Medical Research was one frequently cited example. Mao, then, appears to have been
reacting not only to the content of research but
also to the people making such policy. What could
constitute meaningful regulation of medical research
remained undefined.

The concentration of effort on urban hospitals
drew the bulk of Mao's wrath. The Chairman made
two observations: One, county hospitals were
getting short-changed relative to upper-level
hospitals in the allocation of manpower and equipment.[8] Two, curative services could never reach all
ruralites if resources were exclusively concentrated
in county towns. In the 1964 plan,

. . . more than 90 percent of the higher-level
health workers, more than 70 percent of the
middle-level health workers, more than 80 percent of the expenditures were concentrated in
the hsien, and above hsien, cities.[9]

Directly related to these issues was the fact
that retrenchment policies had produced a decline in
the number of rural, collectively operated, medical
clinics, a phenomenon thoroughly discussed in the
preceding chapters. Despite the sound financial and
political reasons for those reductions, however,
once the nadir of the economic crisis had passed,
broader questions of equity and communitarian
values became of concern to Mao.

The final area of the Chairman's concern related
to the fact that cadres and prestigious individuals
received preferential treatment and access to health
facilities. In August 1964, Mao cryptically reacted
to a Ministry report on health insurance for cadres

187

saying, "Peking Hospital is one where there are many doctors and few patients. It is a hospital of lords. It should be opened to all."[10]   Such an observation resonated well with those who sought more favorable terms of access to the system and this provided an important link in the chain of mobilization that was soon to be forged.

As we have consistently noted, those who were not entitled to health insurance or free medical care had to pay for themselves. While such charges no doubt did not reflect all the "real" costs of care, probably no more than 25 percent of the urban population, and virtually none of the rural populace, was exempted from such burdens. If Premier Chou En-lai's 1967 statement on this issue can be assumed to reflect Mao's thinking, the Chairman wanted a program which would reduce the financial burdens upon these sectors, especially the peasantry.

> Premier Chou had more than once personally instructed Ch'ien Hsin-chung that . . . the current irrational system of medical treatment at public expense should be improved, a part of the appropriation for medical treatment at public expense should be set aside to solve the problem of medical attention to the poor and lower-middle peasants. . . .[11]

The details of such a proposal were never made public. Indeed, they might not have been worked out.

Questions concerning the conditions of physician employment really amounted to a fear that political values were being strangled by the increasing professionalization of the Party itself. Early 1960s patterns of Party recruitment, as we have seen, emphasized physician membership. The Ministry hierarchy was almost exclusively composed of Party members who were simultaneously medical professionals. As has been the case in specialized departments under the Soviet Central Committee and in the Soviet ministries, Party men, who were above all technical specialists, dominated.[12] The Party, at least in the health field, had become the major path for achieving upward mobility, not the major infuser of "Mao's" values.[13]

Mao's evaluation of traditional medicine is relatively opaque because the June 26th statement failed to mention the subject. Chung-i never became a vortex about which Cultural Revolution controversies swirled. While speculative, Mao may have come to believe that stratification within the traditional

Chinese medical profession was similar to that characteristic of western-style practitioners. In a way, the Leap had succeeded too well in creating an independent institutional research and educational base for Chung-i. The elite of the traditional medical community had no more interest in going to the countryside than western-style doctors did.

It is the same thing with herbalists. Ever since counter-revolutionary revisionist Kuo Tzu-hua took charge of the department [the Chung-i-szu], he has placed the whole weight on nine research bases in the country . . . ignoring the serious lack of doctors and medicine in the rural villages.[14]

While Mao had called for renewal of mass health campaigns in 1964, his June 26th statement made no mention of them. Possibly one reason for not mentioning them was that opposition to them was so strong among those he was seeking to mobilize over other issues that to bring up the subject ran the risk of alienating those he would soon need. Given the absence of large-scale mass campaigns (like those of the Leap) in the post-Cultural Revolution period, one assumes that resistance to any new large-scale campaigns is still substantial and that the immediate needs for increased agricultural stability and production have been paramount.

To conclude, the Chairman perceived two fundamentally negative trends in health care, problems which were by no means unique to that realm. First, he saw the emergence of what John W. Lewis has called a "city-to-city system." There was a self-reinforcing quality to this system, with doctors, researchers, local cadres, and political leaders all having a common interest in helping "high quality" facilities in the cities. Because the major institutions for which the health bureaucracy had responsibility were in urban areas, it was these areas which set the bureaucratic agenda. The second trend of concern to Mao was the transformation of the Party. The Chairman faced a supreme dilemma—how to stop the differentiation of ideology while promoting the technological modernization which was requiring increased specialization and division of labor in the society and polity at large. Mao wanted a complex, industrially sophisticated society without the complex and differentiated men needed to staff it.

On the eve of the Cultural Revolution, the Wei-sheng-pu leadership was composed of Ch'ien Hsin-chung (a doctor), Tsui I-t'ien (a doctor), Ho Piao (a doctor), Shih Shu-han (a doctor), Chang Kai (profession unknown), and Kuo Tzu-hua (a traditional practitioner). This predominance of professionals would lead one to expect that such a policy-making body would have a substantially different perspective than Mao, and indeed it did.

Huang Chia-ssu, head of the Chinese Academy of Medical Sciences (a semi-autonomous unit of the Ministry), clearly defined the problems in medical education and health delivery in rural areas as he saw them. Mao's June 26th blast appears to have been a direct and public response to Huang's position.

> . . . many concrete problems also needed to be solved. For example, what is the aim of fostering students . . .? How long is the term of study? What are the entrance requirements for a student? What should be taught? How should lessons be taught? . . . There are insufficient medical personnel, and the State cannot possibly assign many medical doctors to the countryside. . . . The target of fostering cannot be too high, otherwise it may need a very long period of time and a great deal of expense. Neither can the target be too low, otherwise the rural doctors cannot solve questions which ordinary medical workers . . . cannot solve. . . . With regard to the cultural level of students for admission to the medical class, we want junior [sic, senior] middle school graduates.[15]

For Huang, the problem of "whom" to serve had to be seen along with the questions of who should do the serving and how? For what kind of work are doctors to be trained? Insufficient knowledge would render them useless and erode public confidence and over-training would waste scarce resources. If doctors were removed from the cities, who would take care of the already dissatisfied patients there? Admitting "unqualified" students would ultimately satisfy neither teachers, patients, nor students. Most basically, who was going to pay for all of this? These were not the difficulties Mao identified but they were the central problems from the Ministry's perspective.

These concerns were shared by the vice-ministers of health. Hsu Yun-pei had observed, for instance, that "There should not be any shortening of the course. Nor should it be stipulated that a five-year course is to be finished in three years, to free us from the cramping effect. Since most things in the original curriculum should still be retained, . . . how can the number of academic years be reduced?"[16] As late as March 1966, Vice-Minister Chang Kai observed," . . . we must continue our efforts to improve existing five-year or six-year medical colleges, and, at the same time, give medical training in a variety of ways. . . . Our medical schools are organizing short courses to train doctors for rural commune clinics."[17] These views resonated well with Lu Ting-i, the head of the Party's Propaganda and Education Department, who felt that technical skills should not be forgotten in the drive for expansion of the manpower base.[18] Indeed, Mao had agreed with the need for a "varied approach" in February 1964, as noted earlier.

In medical education policy, shared values linked the medical profession (e.g., Huang Chia-ssu), the Ministry (e.g., Hsu Yun-pei and Chang Kai), and those functional divisions of the Party Center most concerned with education (e.g., the Propaganda Department and Lu Ting-i). While each of these levels in the system were internally complex and fragmented themselves, all three sectors agreed that medical education required significant length. By 1965, despite his earlier statements, Mao had locked horns with the professionals.

Ministry and professional perceptions of the problems in medical research diverged from Mao's as well. Huang Chia-ssu articulated the apparent view of most doctors and the Ministry in responding to the Chairman's June 26th blast.

> We are going to concentrate our strength on developing research related to the often seen and common ailments, because this is what affects the greatest number of people, and at the same time we also must give great attention to the research of complex diseases like tumors, heart disease, and hereditary diseases.[19]

Because the masses suffered from complex and difficult diseases, such research was necessary and correct. Researchers and doctors were not enthusiastic about being transferred to small health centers in county towns and rural areas either.

191

I think that if such a doctor is kept in the
big urban hospital, he can play a far greater
role. I secretly worry for doctors like this
and especially the veteran ones or the professors. Are they not being hampered in their
effort toward better scientific research work?[20]

Similarly, Ministry leaders believed that more,
rather than less, research was needed. As Hsu Yun-
pei noted, "The presently existing difficulties are
not problems in the Health Services Bureau of Peking
Hospital, they are [a result] of insufficient concern, understanding, and research in health
work. . . ."[21] Minister of Public Health Ch'ien
Hsin-chung noted that "proceeding with the mass
orientation [of research] superficially tends toward
the workers and the peasants and has world-wide significance. . . . However, in fact, to have world-
wide significance [we] certainly must . . . raise
the standard, promote the pinnacles."[22] The substantial overlap between professional and Ministry
perceptions is apparent; in many respects they were
indistinguishable.

The shape of the health delivery system was an
equally divisive issue. In contrast to Mao's call
for "putting the stress on the rural areas," Vice-
Minister Chang Kai asserted,

From a practical point of view, strengthening
rural health work means to meet the medical
service needs of the peasants, to improve rural
health conditions and provide the material conditions needed for the building of new, socialist villages. From the long-term view, it is
to gradually diminish the differences between
town and country, between industry and agriculture and between mental and manual labor,
prevent the growth of revisionism and carry
the socialist revolution through to the end.[23]

Mao was looking at indicators of rural-urban inequality such as the site of physician residence,
budgetary allocations to various levels of the
system, and the location of facilities. Along
these dimensions, the inequalities were substantial.
The Ministry argued, however, that the real question was, how well are peasant needs being met?
From this perspective, the problem was how to make
the urban hospital system more responsive to peasant
needs? Only in the future could other forms of
inequality be reduced.

Of equal concern to the Ministry was the inequality, and poor quality, of services provided
urbanites. When patients confronted doctors, unions
and the Party expanded the numbers entitled to free
or insured health care, and political figures like
P'eng Chen demanded better services, these were the
demands which were most clearly heard. Minister
Ch'ien observed in August 1965,

> When serving the cities, they have also failed
> to serve satisfactorily the majority of the
> urban population who have been unable to get
> medical assistance.[24]

Ch'ien concluded by saying, ". . . from now on the
focal point of public health work should be placed
not only on the rural villages but also on the
cities without prejudice to each other."[25]
The primary fear of health bureaucrats was that
transfer of health personnel from the cities would
produce a further deterioration in the hospital
system.

> At present the workload of some urban hospitals,
> particularly the big and medium-sized ones, is
> comparatively heavy. If appropriate measures
> cannot keep pace with the requirements of work
> after a relatively large number of medical
> workers are transferred to rural areas, medical
> work will be affected. . . . According to our
> observations, there are many causes for the
> relatively heavy workload in the case of some
> big and medium hospitals in urban areas.[26]

In short, the Wei-sheng-pu held that health work had
to be consolidated in the cities before expansion
into the countryside occurred on a large scale.
People's Daily concluded, "Fundamental reforms are
necessary before urban hospitals will be able to
transfer more medical personnel to rural
areas. . . ."[27]
It appears, from very limited data, that municipal leaders were equally adamant about maintaining
existent levels of urban medical care. P'eng Chen
is said to have informed Minister Ch'ien Hsin-chung:
"The work of the Public Health Ministry reflects
the situation in the great revolution. Priority
must be given to making urban health work a success.
Only after the cities have been put in order in
this respect can we proceed to work the rural villages."[28] Once again, a great commonality of

193

interest between the bureaucracy, urban leaders, and doctors is apparent.

While specific central leaders (e.g., P'eng Chen, Lu Ting-i, and Teng Hsiao-p'ing), the Wei-sheng-pu leadership, and municipal authorities agreed on broad issues such as educational and health care delivery philosophy, other questions, especially financing, tended to divide them. From the viewpoint of the Ministry, expansion of health services required more money. Leaders at the Center who were responsible for making allocations to the entire galaxy of government agencies, however, faced many more requests than they were able to satisfy. Consequently, central leaders, especially Teng Hsiao-p'ing, were often forced to deny funding to programs which they may have actually favored in the abstract. For instance, Minister of Public Health Ch'ien Hsin-chung asked Teng to increase the Ministry's budget so that changes in the health financing system could be made and benefits provided to more people.

> . . . the Ministry of Public Health planned to change the scale of differentiating charges to be paid by the masses for medical treatment and in the plan it asked for an increase in appro-priation. But Ch'ien Hsin-chung first of all approached Teng Hsiao-p'ing for instructions. Teng said to Ch'ien: "You cannot do what you have planned to do; otherwise, my five-year plan will have to be changed too."[29]

The Minister must have felt that his organization was being given constantly expanding responsibili-ties without concomitant increases in resources.

From Teng Hsiao-p'ing's vantage point, the problems were somewhat different. Similar demands for budget increases were probably being made by many other agencies. If he increased the Wei-sheng-pu's budget he would be forced to reduce other allo-cations, increase tax revenues, run a deficit, or reduce the size of any surplus which may have existed. Almost all of these options would have involved the Center in a nightmare of reformulating the budget. Additionally, looking at the experience of the 1950s, one would have concluded that any reduction in medical charges greatly expands demand.

The Ministry saw a further problem in the financing realm. The communes did not appear to be financially vigorous enough to support collective health facilities. "Ch'ien is said to have opposed the rural clinics because they only 'increased the burden' of the communes."[30] From the Wei-sheng-pu's perspective, the county was the only potentially stable financial and administrative unit anywhere near the peasants. The counties, however, had insufficient resources to subsidize commune health centers directly and it was far from clear that commune leaders were interested in reassuming the financial burdens of collective health care. In fact, with the continued emphasis on increasing agricultural production, local leaders would have been loath to rekindle a program that had been associated with previous declines in output. Equally important is the fact that relatively prosperous peasants appear to have believed that the gains to be had from any rural health system that could be established did not justify the expense. In short, central demands for increased production, Wei-sheng-pu predispositions, local fears, and financial constraints all tended to reinforce the policy of making the county hospital the hub of the health system.

Operating within this set of financial and political constraints, the Ministry tried to make county hospitals serve the peasants better by attempting to reduce waste,[31] working county health personnel harder, and trying to improve the system of referral from rural areas. While there are no data to support or refute the proposition, such a policy would be likely to increase the level of conflict between lower and higher levels of the health system, with local units feeling that they were being overworked and underfunded, and higher levels feeling that local units were insufficiently responsive. What role these normal bureaucratic tensions played in the Cultural Revolution is difficult to accurately assess.

The Wei-sheng-pu was confronted with a whole panorama of difficulties relating to the conditions of physician employment. The first was, how could sufficient numbers of urban doctors go to county hospitals without destroying the morale of the physicians and institutions involved, and without depleting already overburdened urban staffs? In February 1965, the first major group of urban physicians was sent to the countryside under the leadership of Huang Chia-ssu. Physicians on such teams felt that their skills were not being maximally utilized in the spartan rural context. One doctor asked, "What did high-grade medical workers do in rural areas? . . . We found ourselves helpless in

195

coping with peasants' demands for medical attention."[32]

The need to designate personnel to go to rural areas proved highly divisive and eroded morale in urban facilities. One hospital, for which data on this point exist, was negatively affected when such decisions had to be made. Each staff member argued why he or she should not go and someone else should.[33] The problems this posed for local health administrators led them to seek the lines of least resistance. The resultant policy (1965-1966) was a compromise; temporary, short-term, transfer of medical personnel to rural areas on a rotating basis, involving as few individuals as possible.

The other major problem confronting the Ministry was the question of how "revolutionarily" to evaluate physician performance without destroying the doctor's incentive or ability to perform? Ministry and professional leaders wanted, at all costs, to avoid a repetition of the Great Leap experience in which political standards had eroded the authority of professionals.[34] The general resolution of the difficulty was advanced by Minister Ch'ien. "The 'redness' of natural scientists ought to be apparent in their research work."[35] The political well-being of professional people had to be judged from their daily work.

SUMMARY

We have identified two alternate definitions of the situation in health care: Mao's and the Wei-sheng-pu's. The Chairman's policy options were reflective of the fact that he was most responsive to those segments of the society which he perceived had been bypassed in the developmental process. Conversely, he was least responsive to organization men who brought up the limitations which material and manpower resources imposed. His concern for the peasantry and his distrust of the cities were, of course, characteristics of his political values going back to the mid-1920s. Mao's inclinations were accentuated by his isolation from day-to-day policy-making in the early 1960s.

The health leadership and its allies at the Center were equally constrained by their day-to-day entanglement in the problems and demands which their roles imposed and which powerful Party, urban, and professional "constituencies" reinforced. These obstacles created a situation in which Ministry

196

leaders saw any rapid departure from the status quo as either impossible or dangerous.

Because Mao believed that leadership composition and values were the decisive factors in policy-making, when he found himself in disagreement with the entire range of medical programs, he concluded that those leaders needed to be replaced. The Ministry leadership quite naturally opposed its own removal and the resultant changes in policy. The following chapter documents the Chairman's creation of a coalition to change Ministry leadership and the strategies which the Wei-sheng-pu employed in an attempt to survive. The struggle described in the pages to come was only one small part of a far larger movement revolving around the major questions of social equity, leadership privilege, developmental strategy, and leadership doctrine.

NOTES

1. Mao Tse-tung, "Reply to Comrade Kuo Mo-jo," Ten More Poems of Mao Tse-tung (Hong Kong: Eastern Horizon Press, 1967), p. 20. In this poem Mao indicates that he felt that he was being ignored in much of the policy process.

2. Mao Tse-tung, "Directive on Public Health Work," in Chairman Mao Talks to the People, ed., Stuart Schram (New York: Pantheon, 1974), pp. 232-233.

3. Mao Tse-tung, "Ch'un-chieh T'an-hua Chi-yao" [Minutes of a spring festival chat] (February 13, 1964), Mao Tse-tung Ssu-hsiang Wan-sui [Long live the thought of Mao Tse-tung] (Peking: August, 1969), pp. 461-462; see also, "The Need for Working Class Leadership of Schools as Seen from Chungshan Medical College," San-chün Lien-wei Chan-pao [Three armies joint committee combat bulletin], September 18, 1968, in Survey of the China Mainland Press (hereafter SCMP), no. 4278, p. 9.

4. "China's Khrushchev Resurrected PUMC to Advance Revisionist Line in Education," China's Medicine 12 (1967):891-892.

5. "China's Khrushchev Resurrected PUMC," pp. 891-892; see also, David M. Lampton, Interview File 21 E.

6. "Chairman Mao in Reception Given to Ch'ien [Hsin-chung?] and Chang [Kai?], August 2, 1965," Hsin Jen

Wei [New people's health] (Peking: People's Health Press, 1967), p. 16.

7. David M. Lampton, Interview File 21 E; see also, Ezra Vogel, Interview No. 42; see also, Ch'üan-wu-ti [Invincible], no. 14.

8. "Fan-ko-ming Hsiu-cheng-chu-i Fen-tzu Ch'ien Hsin-chung Te Chou-ou Li-shih" [The Ugly history of counter-revolutionary revisionist Ch'ien Hsin-chung], Ch'üan-wu-ti [Invincible], no. 14; see also, Hung-i Chan-pao, Pa I Pa Chan-pao [Red medical combat bulletin, August 18 combat bulletin] (June 26, 1967), in Survey of the China Mainland Press-Supplement (hereafter SCMP-S), no. 198; see also, David M. Lampton, Interview File 21 E.

9. Ch'üan-wu-ti [Invincible], no. 17.

10. Mao Tse-tung, "Chairman Mao's Instruction Concerning a Report on the Question of Health Insurance for Senior Cadres Filed by the Party Organization of the Ministry of Health," Hsin Jen Wei, p. 13.

11. "Mayflies Lightly Plot to Topple Giant Tree," Ch'üan-wu-ti [Invincible], no. 17, in SCMP-S, no. 209, p. 19.

12. Jerry Hough, "The Party Apparatchiki," Interest Groups in Soviet Politics, eds., Gordon Skilling and Franklyn Griffiths (Princeton: Princeton University Press, 1971), p. 55.

13. For this argument applied to a broader range of issues see, Michel Oksenberg, "Getting Ahead and Along in Communist China: The Ladder of Success on the Eve of the Cultural Revolution," Party Leadership and Revolutionary Power in China, ed., John W. Lewis (New York: Cambridge University Press, 1970), pp. 304-347.

14. Hung-i Chan-pao, Pa I Pa Chan-pao, p. 32.

15. Huang Chia-ssu, "We Are Confident of Running Part-Farming Part-Study Medical Class," Kuang-ming Jih-pao [Bright daily], May 11, 1965, in SCMP, no. 3471, p. 6.

16. Hung-i Chan-pao, Pa I Pa Chan-pao, pp. 33-34.

17. Chang Kai, "Health Work Serving the Peasants," Chinese Medical Journal 85 (1966):146.

18. Hung-i Chan-pao, Pa I Pa Chan-pao, p. 34.

19. "Huang Chia-ssu Talks About the Achievements of Pharmaceutical and Medical Work," Chung-kuo Hsin-wen [China news], April 5, 1966. Emphasis added.

20. Yeh Yung, "What There is to Gain or Lose is 50-50," SCMP, no. 3591, p. 7.

21. Ch'üan-wu-ti [Invincible], no. 16.

22. Ch'üan-wu-ti [Invincible], no. 14, p. 2.

23. Chang Kai, p. 144. Emphasis added.

24. "Mayflies Lightly Plot to Topple Giant Tree," p. 16.

25. "Mayflies Lightly Plot to Topple Giant Tree," p. 16.

26. "The Direction for Revolutionizing Urban Hospitals," Jen-min Jih-pao [People's daily], September 5, 1965, in SCMP, no. 3547, p. 5.

27. "The Direction for Revolutionizing Urban Hospitals," p. 7. The policy of revolutionizing the city first was rejected in the Cultural Revolution. Kuang-ming Jih-pao [Bright daily], February 7, 1969, noted that this policy had "produced the grave phenomena of rural deficiencies of medicine and drugs."

28. "Mayflies Lightly Plot to Topple Giant Tree," p. 22.

29. "Mayflies Lightly Plot to Topple Giant Tree," p. 21.

30. "The Mao-Liu Controversy Over Rural Public Health," Current Scene 7, no. 12 (1969):6.

31. "Tui-tai Kung-fei I-liao Che Shih Tsen-ma T'ai-tu?" [With what attitude should we treat free medical care?], Hsin-min Wan-pao [New people's evening news], January 11, 1965.

32. "Giving a Prominent Place to Politics and Consciously Making Revolution," Wen-hui Pao, May 20, 1965.

33. David M. Lampton, Interview File 21 E.

34. David M. Lampton, Interview File 21 E. This protocol synopsizes an informant's conversation with a high official of the Chinese Medical Association. This official vowed never to tolerate turmoil of the type witnessed during the Great Leap Forward.

35. "Fan-ko-ming Hsiu-cheng-chu-i Fen-tzu Ch'ien Hsin-chung Te Chou-ou Li-shih," p. 2.

Chapter 9
ASSAULT ON THE HEALTH SYSTEM: STRATEGIES OF POLITICAL OFFENSE AND DEFENSE (AUGUST 1966-1969)

<u>INTRODUCTION</u>

By August 1966, with the publication of the "Sixteen Points" launching the Great Proletarian Cultural Revolution, Mao had reached the conclusion that meaningful policy change required alterations in leadership at the highest levels. During 1965 and the first half of 1966, the Chairman had locked horns with major Party and government figures over several issues, only one of which concerned medical care.

Throughout the late 1965 and early 1966 period, Mao had been unable to get the Peking Mayor (and politburo member), P'eng Chen, to repudiate his literary subordinates who had journalistically attacked the Chairman for the failures of the Great Leap Forward and the subsequent purge of Minister of Defense P'eng Teh-huai. This debate came to a head in May 1966 at an "enlarged" (irregularly constituted) meeting of the Politburo at which P'eng was condemned for his attempts to protect those subordinates. Equally ominous, Director of Propaganda Lu Ting-i was linked to P'eng Chen, although no documents were made public on this in May.[1]

At the same time, throughout much of 1965 Mao faced a protracted debate with Army Chief of Staff Lo Jui-ch'ing over such fundamental issues as: What posture should be adopted with respect to the Soviet Union in the face of American escalation in Vietnam? What were American intentions in Vietnam and what implications did these have for attempts to rectify the Chinese Communist Party? What kind of military was needed to cope with what kinds of threats?[2] Lo argued that American intentions were probably hostile and that military preparedness and modernization had to be the major priorities. This debate ended, like the one involving P'eng Chen, in Mao's triumph. Lo was attacked for his positions in a March 1966 Central Committee Work Group; on March 18th, Lo unsuccessfully attempted to kill himself. At the May 1966 enlarged meeting of the Politburo, Lo was suspended from his posts in the Party and the government.

By late May 1966, students in the major universities began to launch increasingly far-reaching attacks against educators and administrators who either allegedly had ties to the "bourgeois authorities" that had been dealt with earlier in the month or had pursued "revisionist" educational policies themselves. In response, the Party Center (with Chairman Mao in the provinces) sent "work teams" to the schools to guide the rapidly expanding movement. As these work teams sought to guide the movement throughout June and July, they became the targets of attack. Students asserted that the teams were attempting to channel the entire movement in harmless directions. In late July, at Mao's insistence, the work teams were withdrawn. In this atmosphere of tumult, Mao convened an "enlarged" Plenum of the Central Committee which launched the Cultural Revolution. Attack was directed against ". . . those persons in authority who are taking the capitalist road. . . ."[3]

The Cultural Revolution of 1966-1969 was a massive movement in which what was at stake varied according to one's organizational affiliation, values, and interests. Consequently, the campaign defies facile description. Because this study limits its gaze to health care, the reader might incorrectly infer that medicine was the hub around which all of the period's controversies revolved; this was not the case. The urban bias of the medical system was only part of a larger phenomenon of pervasive urban-rural inequalities. The privileged position of cadres in obtaining medical care was only part of the reality of cadre privilege. Finally, professionalism in the Party was widespread and was not confined to the medical system. In brief, health care was not the focal point of the Cultural Revolution, it was merely a policy area in which several fundamental issues intersected. This intersection makes medicine an analytically important subject. Below, we shall examine the strategies which medical bureaucrats, educators, and doctors employed in their attempts to protect themselves and their policies and we shall analyze the strategies which disaffected groups used in their attempts to change such policies and oust such individuals.

MAO'S COALITION BUILDING RESOURCES

The Chairman explicitly sought to create public opinion against the educational structure and the bureaucracy and to legitimate attacks against both. The "Sixteen Points" of August 1966 declared, "To overthrow a political power, it is always necessary, first of all, to create public opinion. . . ."[4] Once the educators and the bureaucrats had been singled out as the bête noire (the bureaucracy was so designated slightly later than the educational system), there was no shortage of individuals to attack the system. Who were these people, how were they mobilized, and what were their objectives?

Rising standards for scholastic performance and reduced enrollments in medical schools during the previous period had meant that many students found it impossible to get into medical school, or stay once they had.[5] ". . . one-third of the students of worker and peasant origin enrolled in 1958 (for the premedical course at Peking University), were thrown out within two years. . . ."[6] Medical school teachers and students who were interviewed agreed that it was these persons who were generally most vociferous in their denunciation of the medical education system.

> The ones [students] who led the Cultural Revolution [in the hospitals and schools] where she was were predominantly the poor students who felt that the basis of their problems was the discrimination of the teacher against workers and peasants.

> The most radical ones, and invariably the worst ones, were the ones who had not made it and were looking for an excuse. . . .[7]

A student interviewee explained that the Red Guards who attacked the administration at Chungshan Medical College in Canton were "the disaffected elements . . . who had not progressed. . . ."[8]

Restricted mobility, for even good students, provided Mao with another reservoir of hostility. Almost all analysts of the mobility situation in China at this time[9] agree that the Youth League and the Party were unable to absorb and advance all

those who wished to get in. Two problems were particularly upsetting to students who could not get
into the Party. First, skilled physicians more
frequently gained admittance than those who lacked
such ability. Secondly, the rewards for being in
the Party were greater than ever before. Students
realized that assignment to desired posts was frequently made on the basis of Party membership.[10]
Quite predictably, when the Cultural Revolution
polarization occurred, those students who were in
the Party or Youth League were generally opposed to
those students who were attacking the school administration, the Party, and the bureaucracy.[11]

Students were not the only sectors of the
polity which Mao could mobilize against hospital and
school administrations; there were traditional doctors, ancillary personnel, and nurses. While traditional doctors sought to insulate themselves from
the turmoil as best they could, in many cases these
practitioners were hostile toward western-style
physicians who had accorded them little deference in
the past. Such persons were often willing to join
the "revolutionary vanguard."[12] There were sound
tactical reasons for traditional doctors to attack
western-style physicians as well. In a struggle as
complex as the Cultural Revolution, the best defense
was a good offense. Equally available for mobilization were many of the ancillary staff and nursing
personnel who (interviewees report) felt that their
importance had been diminished by retrenchment policies. They had been subordinated to medical doctors
in the attempt to reestablish "order" in the post-
Great Leap period. The doctor-nurse relationship is
a tension-laden tie in most countries and Mao tapped
these rather normal discontents.

There were other segments of the urban population which could, and did, attack the health system
directly; contract, temporary, and part-time laborers. As Premier Chou noted in February 1968, "Those
who receive free medical care in the cities are also
a minority . . . the workers are one dividing into
two" (kung-jen chieh-chi i fen-wei-erh).[13] As one
interviewee explained,

> . . . these workers were terribly unhappy over
> the course of events and their livelihood, but
> during the period of anarchism in XX Medical
> College, for instance, temporary and contract
> workers in the hospital did organize and did
> get free medical care for a brief period of
> time . . . they took the hospital chop and

with this they could do whatever they
wanted. . . .[14]

John W. Lewis has described the conflicts of
interest between regular and irregular members of
the work force.[15] The existence of a pool of cheap
labor gave factory managers the chance to lower labor
costs and make regular workers more docile through
threats of replacement. Equally important, irregular workers received few, if any, of the fringe benefits to which regular workers were entitled. While
conflicts of interest between regular and irregular
workers were certainly present, some regular workers
were in a position similar to that of temporary,
part-time, and contract laborers. Regular workers
received far from uniform benefits and their dependents never received comprehensive medical coverage.
Also, even if health financing presented no problem
to such workers, other aspects of the medical system
proved highly abrasive.

One source of discontent was that Ministry and
local health administrators, in an effort to control
costs and waste, had tightened up referral practices,
hoping to weed out "frivolous" cases. While there
were sound reasons for this policy, it further escalated the general level of aggravation with the health
system. Even if a worker did get into the hospital
system he frequently did not receive the kind of
treatment he felt appropriate. One common accusa-
tion was that doctors saved the effective (and scarce)
drugs for cadres.[16] The physical amenities available to elite personages were always relatively substantial. Finally, doctors had to approve requests
for medical leaves of absence and this proved to be
a frequent point of contention between physicians
and workers.[17] In short, health administrators, by
allocating scarce services, attempting to reduce
waste, and responding to the demands of the powerful,
succeeded in alienating vast sectors of the society,
even though it is indisputable that the society was
light years ahead of where it had been in 1949.

Sectors of the peasantry were candidates for mobilization as well.[18] Ruralites on the outskirts of
Shanghai asked, "Why are all the big hospitals and
medical services concentrated in the town? We country-
folk, who have only the mobile medical services, also
have to pay for all medical attention."[19] These
grievances (usually among those persons living in
proximity to urban centers) were consciously manipu-
lated by contending groups in the cities. In many
cases, suburban ruralites (or worker-peasants) joined in

the urban demonstrations, denouncing, and upon occasion beating, doctors and health administrators. One Red Guard explained,

> . . . the peasants in the area of Canton were very unhappy with the general pre-Cultural Revolution health situation in that they had to give deposits before they could enter a county hospital. Also, he said, he knew they were aware that, in the city, people were insured and they were not . . . the amount of yao fei [drug charge] varied, being the highest from 1960-1965; this upset the peasants.[20]

One should not exaggerate the role peasants played generally, and the activism of remote ruralites particularly.[21] The reasons for relatively low levels of peasant involvement are several: (1) Poor rural communications reduced the capacity of peasants to know about, and participate in, urban activities. (2) Because remote inhabitants had less contact with the cities, they presumably experienced less contrast between their life styles and those of the city dweller. (3) Agricultural chores left peasants with little time to participate in distant political activities, and the regime wanted minimal disruption of agricultural production.[22] One informant explained,

> . . . basically the people in the cities were more aware of the nation as a totality and the effect that central policies would have on them but that peasants weren't really in the nation as much as they were in the communes . . . the health of the commune was much more salient to them than some more abstract national policy.[23]

With those sectors of the society identified above constituting the core of Mao's coalition, educational institutions became the focus of conflict through December 1966. In January 1967, the struggle moved into the "seize power" phase and the primary target of attack became the Wei-sheng-pu specifically, and the bureaucracy, generally. With the public encouragement of Mao's wife, Chiang Ch'ing, and Defense Minister Lin Piao, "Red Rebels" appeared in the major ministries.[24] Who were these individuals and what motivated them to confront their superiors?

First of all, the fact that many top bureaucrats had occupied the same posts for years on end created

a situation in which middle and lower-level functionaries had poor expectations for upward mobility.[25] The Wei-sheng-pu had had an especially
stable leadership since the mid-1950s. Those few
positions which had opened up had been filled with
men just as senior as the ones they replaced (e.g.,
Shih Shu-han and Ch'ien Hsin-chung).

> . . . many lower-level bureaucrats did defect
> [from their superiors] in the Cultural Revolu-
> tion and the . . . explanation lies in the
> nature of bureaucratic antagonisms gener-
> ally. . . .[26]

Another source of antagonism within the Ministry of Public Health was interdepartmental friction,
a subject about which we know relatively little.
For example, local public health bureaus have traditionally been vociferous in attacking the curative
biases of the Ministry's Education Bureau.[27] Also,
one would anticipate that local health bureaus which
had been given continually expanding responsibilities and slowly expanding resources would have felt
hostility toward those bureaucrats they held responsible for that situation. Finally, one would expect
that the lean budgets of the early 1960s had exacerbated tensions.

The final motive for bureaucratic subordinates
to attack their superiors relates to the bureaucrat's need for stability and security. By December
1966, local medical and educational facilities were
in disarray, funding proposals were probably lan-
guishing, and there was uncertainty over the direction in which to move. In November it had been
announced that schools would remain closed for a
year. In stark terms, Ministry leaders had lost
much of their utility to subordinates. They provided neither security nor predictability. Secondly,
in the context of Mao's June 26, 1965 blast, it was
obvious that the pinnacles of the Wei-sheng-pu were
vulnerable.

> Once an individual bureaucrat's loyalty to Mao
> was questioned . . . his power--based upon his
> network of friends, his control over informa-
> tion, and the allocation of his limited
> resources--gradually eroded. Other bureaucrats
> sought to disassociate themselves from
> him. . . .[28]

One should keep in mind that those who first identified and attacked "renegades" would subsequently be

less vulnerable to charges of complicity themselves.

In short, the level of threat was high and the security of the leadership tenuous. When the Cultural Revolution was extended to the Ministry in late 1966 and early 1967, middle and lower-level bureaucrats were scared. These kinds of personal survival decisions led every interviewee who lived through these events to say that the movement was a "power struggle" devoid of policy content.

There existed, then, a symmetry of interests between "revolutionary" medical students, frightened and/or ambitious middle-level bureaucrats, specific sectors of the working population, suburban peasants, and central leaders such as Chiang Ch'ing and Lin Piao. Robinson makes the important observation that even Premier Chou En-lai had an interest in promoting radical takeovers (within limits) once bureaucrats began to practice "economism" and disrupt production.

Middle-level bureaucrats were in a position to inflict great damage on their superiors; they could release documents. One would expect that leaks would have occurred in departments which (a) had sensitive documents and (b) felt most threatened. That is, indeed, where leaks appear to have occurred. Employees in the office of Chien-k'ang Pao (Health bulletin) and the Health Services Bureau (Pao-chien-chü) took the leading role in releasing Wei-sheng-pu files. The vehicle for disseminating these documents was Ch'üan-wu-ti (Invincible), a tabloid compiled and distributed by functionaries of the Chien-k'ang Pao and the Health Services Bureau.[29] These organizations were particularly vulnerable because Chien-k'ang Pao had been the mouthpiece of the Ministry's Party Committee and Mao had called for abolition of the Health Services Bureau in August 1964.[30] In addition to these Red Rebel groups, there was an entire constellation of other organizations inside and outside the Ministry which attacked "power-holders." While we have the names of these groups, we know little about their composition or leadership (See Appendix C).

In sum, two kinds of groups were most active in denouncing the Ministry's leadership: (a) Those individuals within the bureaucracy that felt most threatened and (b) those persons who had suffered most during the retrenchment phase. This was a situation ripe for coalition politics.

The situation confronting the Ministry went
through three distinct phases: the June 1965-June
1966 period, the June 1966-January 1967 period, and
the January 1967-August 1967 period. In the 1965-
1966 phase, the problem facing the leadership was
how to deal with Mao's demands for reform and,
simultaneously, avoid aggravating all of the difficulties which the Ministry perceived it already
faced. From June 1966-December 1966, the objective
was to confine and limit the disturbances in the
schools and medical centers. In the January-August
1967 phase, the question was survival of the health
leadership itself. The resources necessary to accomplish one task were not the same as those required
for success at another. In the final analysis, the
value of Wei-sheng-pu resources progressively
declined.

The June 1965-June 1966 period. The Ministry's
major resource was policy-making discretion in the
face of a vague directive. Mao's June 26th blast
was sufficiently unspecific that the Ministry could
give it substance in a variety of ways. The bureaucracy could establish the order in which goals were
to be achieved and allocate resources. The best
way to illustrate the Ministry's capacities in this
regard is to identify twelve "strategies" which it
employed in attempting to maximize its control and
minimize the disruption which it feared Mao's proposals would create.

(1) The Ministry could define who "the masses"
were and what they wanted. For instance, in his
June 26th directive, Mao had called for greater
attention to ". . . the problems to which the masses
most need solutions."[31] Minister of Public Health
Ch'ien Hsin-chung is supposed to have replied,
"Making science and medicine mass in character, on
the face of it, tends toward the workers, peasants,
soldiers . . . however, in reality the masses want
to raise the level, want the pinnacles."[32] Additionally, the Ministry could broaden the definition
of "the masses" thereby leaving itself the freedom
to focus on aspects of policy most compatible with
its own predispositions and resources. For instance,
Minister Ch'ien made a speech shortly after Mao's in
which he said, "When serving the cities, they have
also failed to serve satisfactorily the majority of
the urban population who have been unable to get
medical assistance."[33]

(2) The second strategy was to admit to more
errors than accused of, many minor in nature, and then
"solve" those. This tactic was used extensively.
Ch'ien countered the Chairman by asserting that there
had been two basic problems with Ministry work: (a)
There had been too little democracy and (b) too much
bureaucracy. The Minister told the Ministry Party
Committee that, "It is meaningless to write those
things. Several reports we made previously talked
about democracy; we should concentrate on this
issue."[34] In short, bureaucrats could multiply the
problems with which policy had to cope, thereby giving
themselves the opportunity to select the targets.

(3) Strategy three involved redefining the "primary contradiction." Mao's critique of the Ministry
boiled down to the assertion that rural-urban inequality was the fundamental problem. Ch'ien employed
the strategy of redefining the "primary contradiction"
in his August 1965 address to the National Conference on Rural Medical Education and thereafter. He
asserted that the major contradiction was "between
man and disease." Similarly, the Minister said that
the problem was not only how to take care of peasants,
but how to take care of peasants and urbanites.[35]

(4) Strategy four involved telling Mao that his
policy would hurt those sectors of the society he
valued most. For instance, regarding paramedic education, the Ministry of Public Health and Lu Ting-i
maintained that if such personnel were insufficiently trained the peasants would be further alienated
and future programs would founder. "The time for
study should not be too short. Don't spoil the brand
[sic. name] of part-farming and part-medical work."[36]
Regarding sending large numbers of medical personnel
to the countryside, in January 1966 Ch'ien cogently
argued, "If everybody goes down to the countryside
and does not make a success of his work, he will
increase the burden of the countryside."[37]

(5) The Ministry sought to make completion of
its policies a precondition for realizing Mao's objectives. A conspicuous example of this tactic was
Liu Shao-ch'i's reported remark, "If there is no good
solution to the revolutionization of the medical
services of the city, there cannot be any good solution to the diversion of the health services to the
rural villages. . . ."[38] Urban leaders such as
Peking Mayor P'eng Chen had a vested interest in this
formulation as well. "Only after the cities have
been put in order . . . can we proceed to work the
rural villages."[39]

(6) The Ministry could set up "model units,"
pump inordinate resources into them, and then

proclaim them a success while assuaging the professionals assigned to them. In August 1965, the Ministry assigned Vice-Minister Tsui I-t'ien to supervise a model in Kiangsu Province, Ho Piao was assigned one in Hupeh, Ch'ien was responsible for the one in Peking's suburban T'ung County, and Chang Chih-ch'iang was to supervise the model in Hunan. These models became a strategy to cope with Mao, rather than tests laying the foundation for nationwide implementation, when the Ministry began to concentrate enormous resources in these "key points" (chung tien). Each vice-minister had a substantial discretionary fund for his center. Tsui I-t'ien, for example, was accused of having tried to divert over one-third of Kiangsu Province's medical equipment and supplies to his one health center in Chujung County.[40] Ch'ien Hsin-chung allegedly outfitted the clinic for which he was responsible with equipment which no ordinary county facility could afford or use.[41]

(7) The Wei-sheng-pu made compliance contingent on larger budgetary allocations. This strategy shifted the onus of failure from the Ministry to those at the Center (e.g., Teng Hsiao-p'ing) who were unable or unwilling to increase health appropriations. As noted earlier, the Ministry had refused to act upon Premier Chou's demands for reform of health financing when Teng Hsiao-p'ing said that increased appropriations were impossible. This strategy made it possible for ministerial bureaucrats to play central leaders off against one another.

(8) The Ministry leadership could protect itself by linking its policies with a sacrosanct organ or personality and by manipulating information which might prove harmful to high-level personalities. Ch'ien employed this strategy in July 1965 by saying, "If we say there are errors in direction, what position does this put the Center in?"[42] For whatever set of reasons, Vice-Premier T'ao Chu was allegedly given responsibility for forestalling attacks on the Wei-sheng-pu. In June 1966, as the tempo of the Cultural Revolution accelerated, T'ao declared there were no "black elements" in the Ministry.[43]

An additional source of Ministry leverage was its possession of sensitive information relating to Lu Ting-i, Teng Hsiao-p'ing, and Liu Shao-ch'i. One documented case of this concerned Lu Ting-i and his wife Yen Wei-ping. Since the early 1960s, Yen apparently had been suffering from mental illness and allegedly wrote hysterical letters to Lin Piao.[44] As Lin's power grew, such letters acquired political significance and Lu wanted to "cover up" the whole

affair. Later charges asserted that Yen's mental
illness was contrived by doctors and Lu in order to
hide Yen's political deviance. Irrespective of Yen's
mental condition, only Ch'ien Hsin-chung, Teng Hsiao-
p'ing, Vice-Minister Shih Shu-han, Vice-Minister
Huang Shu-tse, and Ch'ien's wife (in the Neurology
Department of Peking Hospital) knew anything about
the problem. Concisely, some central leaders had
personal reasons for insulating the Ministry from
attack.

(9) The Ministry, and allies at the Center, had
discretion in determining what organizations would
conduct criticism and how extensively it was to proceed. With persons sympathetic to the Ministry in
control of the central Party apparatus, and the Wei-
sheng-pu Party Committee composed almost exclusively
of medical professionals, there was little danger of
criticism "getting out of hand," if the Party remained the instrument of rectification. On June 25,
1966, T'ao Chu gave the Ministry Party Committee a
clean bill of ideological health and charged it with
leading rectification.

> The current great cultural revolution movement
> must completely be placed under the leadership
> of the Party, because that constitutes a hall-
> mark for drawing a dividing line between the
> genuine and false leftists. Those who want to
> get rid of and oppose the leadership of the
> Party are phony leftists but genuine rightists
> regardless of how high-sounding their slogans
> and how good their features are.[45]

(10) The Ministry could claim that it had expertise which entitled it to authority in specific
policy areas. To advance this argument was probably
a liability in the long-run, but it was employed in
the early stages of the movement. After the Chairman's June 26th directive, Vice-Minister of Public
Health Hsu Yun-pei said that medical education should
not be shortened and then asked, "Since most things
in the original curriculum should still be retained,
. . . how can the number of academic years be
reduced?"[46] Only professionals knew what was
necessary so they should be decisive in determining
curriculum length.

Another report even more boldly projected the
contours of this argument. The question was asked,
"Can politics cure disease?" "Many cadres pointed
out in the debate that politics could never replace
medical science, nor take the place of medicine. A

political instructor, they argued, can teach
Marxism-Leninism but cannot remove a tumor from a
patient's body."[47]

(11) The Ministry flooded lower-level health
units with directives forcing them to set priorities.
After the June 26th directive, the Ministry promoted
a model county hospital which had allegedly reduced
examination and drug costs, increased access to
facilities, and reduced red tape.[48] The Ministry's
leaders must have known that most counties were in
no position to make all these changes simultaneously, yet, by asking they removed some of the onus of
failure from themselves. One side effect of this
strategy was that this exacerbated the tensions
which existed between higher and lower-level units.
Local authorities were not particularly loyal when
the "seize power" phase began.

Additional dangers adhered to this approach.
If lower-level institutions chose unorthodox ways to
solve problems this could become a club with which
to beat the Ministry. This operational independence
provided opponents with much of their ammunition in
the first months of 1967. For example, the Ministry
directed medical facilities to send one-third of
their personnel to rural areas, without precisely
specifying the categories of persons to be involved.
Quite naturally, local authorities tried to hang
onto scarce professional personnel. "Hospitals held
fast to the backbone technical force in their staff
lists. . . . Some units, unable to reach their targets, even resorted to conferring the title of 'doctor' on their administrative personnel. . . . The
personnel were asked to keep this secret from the
peasants."[49]

(12) This approach took the form of saying that
Mao's policy was unclear and more time was needed to
study it. For example, Mao's June 26th directive
said nothing about Chung-i. In trying to keep traditional medicine out of the rapidly escalating discussion, Ch'ien said,

> I don't know what the policy toward Chinese
> medicine is, I only know the policy of combining
> western and Chinese medicine, and therefore
> these few years will be utilized to research
> the union of traditional and western medicine.[50]

LIMITING THE SCOPE OF ATTACK, JUNE 1966-JANUARY 1967

In June and July 1966, the struggle left the
preemptive stage and entered a phase in which

medical schools were disrupted by Red Guards. The problem became how to limit the scope and impact of attacks. Because medical schools were under several different administrative jurisdictions, and local political situations were variable, we shall confine the analysis to two medical schools under central jurisdiction.[51] In these cases it is feasible to link Wei-sheng-pu strategies with local realities.

The first major resource which the Ministry had to use in counteracting student disruptions was T'ao Chu's directive that the Ministry should rely on work teams in the schools, and that the teams should concentrate on "education," not struggle.[52] In both medical schools the work teams became a target of attack in July 1966, with rebellious students asserting that they were designed to manage, not promote, the revolution.[53] With the late July withdrawal of work teams and the August closure of schools (and the November extension of that policy), this strategy collapsed. In short, the Ministry first sought to pull in its organizational net and channel criticism.

The second resource which the Ministry had was the opposition of many students and staff to the disruptive activities of rebels in the medical colleges. Those who had benefitted from the previous policy were highly motivated to maintain the status quo ante. A predictable coalition formed. Students who were doing well and had prospects for urban mobility allied with older professors and physicians, Party members, some hospital and school administrators, upwardly bound student cadres, and the offspring of cadres. This coalition (or confluence of interests) provided the most durable resource which the Wei-sheng-pu had. No high-level purge could eliminate it and its resilience produced prolonged factionalism. In fact, these cleavages have had important political consequences in the 1970s, as we shall see.

THE "SEIZE POWER" PHASE, JANUARY-AUGUST 1967

By the beginning of the "seize power" phase in January 1967, most of the Ministry's major resources had been devalued or neutralized. By December 1966, Liu Shao-ch'i, Teng Hsiao-p'ing, P'eng Chen, Lu Ting-i, and T'ao Chu had all been sacked. The entire fabric of Ministry-Center relationships had been disrupted. Simultaneously, the legitimacy of the Party to control the movement had been undermined

214

by the work team issue and Mao's August call to "bombard the headquarters." Ministry leaders had lost their legitimacy and protection. It was only a matter of time until lower-level bureaucrats "defected." They only needed to be authoritatively told that attacks on the government structure were permissible. On November 3, 1966, Lin Piao did just that.

> The broad masses have really translated into action Chairman Mao's call to "concern yourselves with the affairs of state." . . . By this extensive democracy, the Party is fearlessly permitting the broad masses to . . . supervise the Party and government leading institutions and leaders at all levels.[54]

Premier Chou's move to the left in November and December 1966 removed the last obstacle to attacking the government.[55] The premier only continued to protect those he deemed most important and easily "salvaged," persons such as Vice-Premier Li Hsien-nien. The Ministry was not deemed one of those organizations, and January 1967 marked the beginning of a struggle in the Wei-sheng-pu. What resources did this organization have in this bare knuckles encounter?

Three participants in the Ministry struggle can be identified: the Red Rebels, the Wei-sheng-pu leadership, and the People's Liberation Army (hereafter PLA). The ensuing battle evolved in much the same way as events in the medical schools had. The Ministry employed three resources to counter the opposing coalition: (a) the PLA, (b) loyal subordinates, and (c) the weapon of last resort, obfuscation.

In the last months of 1966 and the first months of 1967, the PLA played a stabilizing (or "conservative") role, as it did throughout society. In September 1966, General Sun Cheng (also deputy director of the Party's Cultural and Education Department) assumed responsibility for rectification in the Ministry.[56] Sun established more than twenty "cadre teams" which were supposed to organize and control the movement within the Ministry. The leader of each team was the head of a Ministry bureau or unit.[57] By March 1967, Sun came under attack for the cadre teams for much the same reasons that "work teams" had been denounced earlier.[58] They were quickly disbanded.

215

In the Ministry, as in the polity at large, the PLA had not acted as a revolutionary catalyst and the central authorities, under the sway of the Cultural Revolution Group, issued the January 23 directive calling for the PLA to "support the left."

The so-called "non-involvement" is false, for the army was already involved long ago. The question, therefore, is not one of involvement or non-involvement. It is one of whose side we should stand on and whether we should support the revolutionaries or the conservatives or even the Rightists.[59]

Once the PLA was given this charge, Sun trotted out his PLA uniform, dusted it off, and put it on. Most functionaries of the health system had thought Sun was functioning in his army capacity all along, although this was not the case. This shift, along with the cadre teams, had the effect of causing February to pass relatively quietly. In March, however, the burgeoning Red Rebel groups began to attack the cadre teams and say that "counter-revolutionary elements" were using Sun.[60] The problem facing the rebels was how to attack all the "capitalist roaders" standing behind Sun without attacking him, and by implication, the PLA.

Simultaneously, a proliferation of Red Rebel groups, and counter-organizations, occurred in response to the increasingly extreme rhetoric of Lin Piao and Chiang Ch'ing. While data on the formation of these groups are spotty, the outlines of the process are clear.

On February 28, 1967, the "Ministry of Health Revolutionary Committee" (Wei-sheng Ko Hui) was established, without approval of the Ministry's leadership. The "Revolutionary Committee," was an umbrella organization subsuming a large, but uncertain, number of Red Rebel groups. The Ministry's leaders apparently felt threatened and within the week set up a counter-organization named the "Preparatory Committee of the Ministry of Public Health Revolutionary Rebel Committee" (Wei-sheng-pu Ko Tsao-fan Wei-yüan-hui Ch'ou-wei-hui).[61] According to the Preparatory Committee's opposition, the "Preparatory Committee" had been established at the behest of the Ministry Party Committee and authorized by Vice-Ministers Chang Kai, Tsui I-t'ien, Ho Piao, and Huang Shu-tse.[62]

The "Preparatory Committee's" two major constituent organizations were "The East is Red" and

216

"Revolutionary Liaison" (Ko Lien). Apparently, the department heads who had led the cadre teams of late 1966 and early 1967 controlled these two groups, in addition to three others.[63] If these charges are correct, by March the Ministry leadership had given up trying to stifle the movement and now sought to confuse the situation by proliferating the number of groups involved.

The struggle between rebel factions continued throughout March with two rebel groups becoming increasingly prominent: "The Chien-k'ang Pao Yenan Commune" and the "Capital Hospital Revolutionary Committee."[64] The "Yenan Commune" was in a particularly strategic position; it had access to sensitive Wei-sheng-pu files.

Because the PLA had not adequately responded to the central directive of January, in April the army was once again ordered to "support the left" and not to use force against the rebels.

> Chairman Mao directs the Chinese PLA to intervene in local great cultural revolutions and give the Left vigorous support. . . . (1) In dealing with mass organizations, be they revolutionary or controlled by reactionary elements, or when their situation is not clear, shooting is forbidden. . . . (2) Arbitrary arrests are forbidden, particularly large-scale arrests. . . . (3) It is forbidden to arbitrarily declare a mass organization a reactionary organization and repress it.[65]

With this directive, the Ministry's dike gave way and the torrent of Red Rebel groups went to work. On May 19, 1967, Invincible, the voice of the "Yenan Commune," released secret files relating to the already mentioned Yen Wei-ping affair.[66] This implicated the Wei-sheng-pu's major figures. At the same time, Sun Cheng was blasted for carrying out the "bourgeois line." The entire top veneer of leadership was undermined. Shortly after this, Premier Chou apparently found it impossible to defend the Ministry and decided to, in Robinson's words, "feed" the hapless individuals to the rebels. In two separate meetings with the Red Rebels (May 28, 1967 and June 1, 1967), Chou tried to legitimize past attacks on the Ministry and to simultaneously lay the framework for ending the factionalism that was becoming increasingly severe.[67]

Quite predictably, after Chou's support was thrown to the rebel cause, Ministry leaders had

virtually no identifiable allies. As a consequence,
June, July, and August were devoted to "beating the
dead tigers." More and more evidence was accumulated to demonstrate the perfidy of Ch'ien Hsin-
chung and his "accomplices."

One indication of the Wei-sheng-pu's vulnerability was the fact that of the fifteen ministers
and twenty-seven vice-ministers still holding office
as of October 1, 1967, none was from the Ministry.[68]
Below this level of highly visible top leadership,
permanent personnel changes do not appear to have
been extensive. This basic continuity of second
echelon leadership has been important in the post-
Cultural Revolution policy-making process. Interviews indicate that the same situation prevailed in
medical schools and other related facilities. In
short, the Cultural Revolution did not clean house,
it only dusted things off a bit.

INTERIM LEADERS APPEAR

With the deactivation of the previous Ministry
leadership, a new group of persons assumed interim
responsibility. Three criteria seemed to have been
used in selecting this leadership: (a) PLA membership for the number one person, (b) anonymity, and
(c) some administrative and medical background.
While the formation of "three-in-one alliances" was
the policy in hospitals and schools, no such apparatus was established in the Ministry itself. Because
"Revolutionary Committees" had been unable to con-
tain factionalism in schools, and because the Wei-
sheng-pu could not afford prolonged division, the
PLA sent new personnel to the Ministry in late 1967
(month uncertain).[69]

Once Sun Cheng had departed from the Ministry,
a PLA lieutenant general named Ch'iu Kuo-kuang took
over the number one spot.[70] Ch'iu's credentials
were few, other than his experience in logistics.
Interviews assert that Ch'iu was not operationally
important and that Hsieh Hua (a physician) was much
more important in this respect.[71] In 1970, Ch'iu
was relieved of his position (for reasons that are
unclear) and Hsieh became an increasingly dominant
force in the Wei-sheng-pu, until the reappearance of
Ch'ien Hsin-chung and Huang Shu-tse in 1973 and
1974, topics to which we shall return in the following chapter.[72]

The identity of the rest of the Ministry leadership was not made public until 1971, when four

individuals emerged as the equivalent of vice-ministers: Chou Fa-yen, Hsing Cheng-chin, Yen Chun, and Ma Ching-fen. Fu I-ch'eng, a respected medical person himself, assumed day-to-day responsibility in the Chinese Medical Association. Huang Chia-ssu was back as head of the Chinese Academy of Medical Sciences by about this time. By 1971, the major hospitals were staffed largely by personalities that had held their positions prior to the Cultural Revolution. Efforts to "get things moving again" forced this interim leadership to fall back on old patterns of authority and expertise. This inevitably favored the previous leadership. The re-emergence of Ch'ien Hsin-chung and Huang Shu-tse in 1973 and 1974 was merely a conspicuous part of this process.

Presently, not enough is known about the 1968-1969 leadership to talk about its propensities, the constraints which it confronted, and the resources at its disposal. The impact of the Cultural Revolution on policy, the long-term impact on leadership, and the costs of those changes, will be the subjects explored in the next chapter.

SUMMARY

The Cultural Revolution was an escalating struggle in which two opposing coalitions faced one another. In the June 1965-June 1966 period, the Chairman defined the issues and the Ministry employed a dozen bureaucratic strategies to minimize the disruption which those proposals entailed. In the June to December 1966 phase, Mao changed the issue to that of power in the medical schools. In escalating the point at issue, he broadened the range of resources upon which he could draw to weld a coalition. The Party apparatus tried to reduce the disruption by sending work teams into the medical schools.

By November 1966, it had become apparent that, if the question of power in the schools was to be resolved, a further escalation in Cultural Revolution objectives was required. With Lin Piao's attacks on the governmental structure, the issue had become state power. In escalating the level of contradiction higher, Mao was able to mobilize still more members to his coalition. Significantly, each escalation put the Ministry in an increasingly disadvantageous position. By defining the issue as power, everyone was permitted to dream about whose hands ought to grasp the authority once it was wrenched from the hands of the common bureaucratic enemy. While this was a useful device to build a coalition, it was not helpful in gaining subsequent consensus on knotty policy issues.

The Cultural Revolution does not appear to have changed leadership composition immediately below the top officials; even at this level the old leadership was reappearing by 1973. The immediate impact of the Cultural Revolution was to remove major policy-making authority from the disorganized Ministry and give it to a small elite at the top. In the 1968-1969 period, then, the explanation for the shape of medical policy had little to do with the Ministry of Public Health. We must look to the polity's pinnacles.

NOTES

1. Edward E. Rice, Mao's Way (Berkeley: University of California Press, 1974), pp. 241-243.

2. Harry Harding and Melvin Gurtov, "The Purge of Lo Jui-ch'ing: The Politics of Chinese Strategic Planning," Rand Paper, no. R-548-PR (1971).

3. "Decision of the Central Committee of the Chinese Communist Party Concerning the Great Proletarian Cultural Revolution," CCP Documents of the Great Proletarian Cultural Revolution 1966-1967 (Hong Kong: Union Research Institute, 1968), p. 42.

4. "Decision of the Central Committee of the Chinese Communist Party Concerning the Great Proletarian Cultural Revolution," p. 42.

5. For more on the education problem see, Neale Hunter, Shanghai Journal (New York: Praeger, 1969); see also, John Gardner, "Educated Youth and Urban-Rural Inequalities, 1958-66," The City in Communist China, ed., John W. Lewis (Stanford: Stanford University Press, 1971), pp. 235-286; see also, John W. Lewis, "Commerce, Education, and Political Development in Tangshan, 1956-69," The City in Communist China, pp. 165-168.

6. "China's Khrushchev Resurrected PUMC to Advance Revisionist Line in Education," China's Medicine 12 (1967):892.

7. David M. Lampton, Interview File 21 E, nos. 1 and 6.

8. David M. Lampton, Interview File 21 G.

9. See, for example, John Israel, "The Red Guards in Historical Perspective: Continuity and Change in the Chinese Youth Movement," China Quarterly, no. 30 (1967), pp. 1-32; see also, James R. Townsend, Politics in China (Boston: Little, Brown, and Company, 1974), pp. 242-274; also, Michel Oksenberg, "Getting Ahead and Along in Communist China: The Ladder of Success on the Eve of the Cultural Revolution," Party Leadership and Revolutionary Power in China, ed., John W. Lewis (London: Cambridge University Press, 1970), pp. 304-347.

10. David M. Lampton, Interview File 21 E. This interviewee noted that she only took on research assistants who were both professionally excellent and Party members. She noted that the pool of those who were qualified was sufficiently large (relative to the number of slots) that there generally was no need to assume political risks in order to obtain quality.

11. David M. Lampton, Interview File 21 G.

12. David M. Lampton, Interview File 21 G.

13. "Chou Tsung-li, Li Hsien-nien Fu-tsung-li Chieh-chien Wei-sheng Hsi-t'ung Yü Kuan Tai-piao Shih Te Chiang-hua" [Premier Chou and Vice-Premier Li Hsien-nien's speech to a meeting of representatives of the health system], Lao-kung Chan-pao [Laboring combat bulletin] (February 3, 1968).

14. David M. Lampton, Interview File 21 E.

15. Lewis, "Commerce, Education, and Political Development in Tangshan, 1956-69," pp. 162-165.

16. Ezra Vogel, Interview No. 35, p. 7.

17. David M. Lampton, Interview File 21 E, no. 4, p. 3.

18. For an excellent discussion of peasants and the Cultural Revolution see, Richard Baum, "The Cultural Revolution in the Countryside: Anatomy of a Limited Rebellion," The Cultural Revolution in China, ed., Thomas Robinson (Berkeley: University of California Press, 1971), pp. 367-476.

19.   "Quarterly Chronicle and Documentation," China Quarterly, no. 30 (1967), p. 207.

20.   David M. Lampton, Interview File 21 G.

21.   Baum, p. 367.   "For most of China's 550 million or more rural peasants and basic-level cadres, most of the time, the Cultural Revolution was simply not a particularly salient fact of everyday life."

22.   Central directives of September 14, 1966, December 15, 1966, February 20, 1967, March 7, 1967, and July 13, 1967 were designed to minimize the impact of the movement on agricultural production.

23.   David M. Lampton, Interview File 21 G, p. 2.

24.   For detail on the expansion of the movement to the government apparatus see, Thomas Robinson, "Chou En-lai and the Cultural Revolution in China," The Cultural Revolution in China, pp. 165-312.

25.   Donald W. Klein, "The State Council and the Cultural Revolution," Party Leadership and Revolutionary Power in China, p. 353.

26.   David M. Lampton, Interview File 21 B.

27.   Chien-k'ang Pao [Health bulletin] (May 7, 1957).

28.   Michel Oksenberg, "Occupational Groups in Chinese Society and the Cultural Revolution," The Cultural Revolution 1967 in Review, Michigan Papers in Chinese Studies, no. 2 (1968), p. 31.

29.   Ch'üan-wu-ti [Invincible] began publication in January 1967 and continued until at least August 1967.   The tabloid was published by the "Capital Hospital Revolutionary Committee" and the "Chien-k'ang Pao Yenan Commune."   The paper carried articles authored by at least seventeen different Red Rebel and Red Guard organizations.   When Chou En-lai encouraged attacks on the Ministry in May and June 1967, he used this paper as his vehicle.

30.   Hsin Jen Wei [New people's health] (Peking: People's Health Press, 1967), p. 13.

31.   Mao Tse-tung, "Directive on Public Health," Chairman Mao Talks to the People, ed., Stuart Schram (New York: Pantheon, 1974), p. 232.

32. Ch'üan-wu-ti [Invincible], no. 14, p. 2.

33. "Mayflies Lightly Plot to Topple Giant Tree,"
Ch'üan-wu-ti [Invincible] (June 26, 1967), in Survey
of the China Mainland Press-Supplement (hereafter
SCMP-S), no. 209, p. 16.

34. "Mayflies Lightly Plot to Topple Giant Tree,"
p. 15.

35. "Mayflies Lightly Plot to Topple Giant Tree,"
p. 16.

36. "Mayflies Lightly Plot to Topple Giant Tree,"
p. 22.

37. "Mayflies Lightly Plot to Topple Giant Tree,"
p. 15.

38. "Monstrous Crimes of Urban Lords' Health Minis-
try in Opposing June 26 Directive," Hung-i Chan-pao,
Pa I Pa Chan-pao [Red medical combat bulletin,
August 18 combat bulletin] (June 26, 1967), in
SCMP-S, no. 190, p. 31.

39. "Mayflies Lightly Plot to Topple Giant Tree,"
p. 22.

40. "Mayflies Lightly Plot to Topple Giant Tree,"
p. 21.

41. "Mayflies Lightly Plot to Topple Giant Tree,"
p. 21.

42. Ch'üan-wu-ti [Invincible], no. 16, p. 3.

43. Ch'üan-wu-ti [Invincible], no. 6, p. 4.

44. "Striking Counter-Revolutionary Case," Ch'üan-
wu-ti [Invincible], no. 9, in SCMP-S, no. 204, p. 8.

45. "T'ao Chu is the Khrushchev of Central-South
China," Current Background (hereafter CB), no. 824,
p. 46.

46. "Monstrous Crimes of Urban Lords' Health Ministry . . .," pp. 33-34.

47. "Can Politics Cure Disease?", China News Summary, no. 113, p. C4.

48. "Fang-pien Nung-min K'an-ping, Chien-ch'ing Nung-min Tze-tan" [Make it more convenient for peasants to receive medical treatment and lighten their burdens], Kuang-ming Jih-pao [Bright daily], October 14, 1965.

49. "Mayflies Lightly Plot to Topple Giant Tree," p. 18.

50. Ch'üan-wu-ti [Invincible], no. 14.

51. David M. Lampton, Interview Files 21 E and 21 G. These interviews provide the basis for this analysis. Both schools were prestigious facilities under direct central control.

52. Ch'üan-wu-ti [Invincible], no. 6, p. 4.

53. David M. Lampton, Interview File 21 G.

54. Peking Review, no. 46 (1966), pp. 10-11.

55. Robinson, "Chou En-lai and the Cultural Revolution in China," pp. 188-191.

56. For more on Sun Cheng see, Who's Who In Communist China (Hong Kong: Union Press, 1970), p. 579; also, David M. Lampton, Interview File 21 E.

57. Ch'üan-wu-ti [Invincible], nos. 6 and 11; see also, David M. Lampton, Interview File 21 E, no. 6.

58. Ch'üan-wu-ti [Invincible], no. 6, p. 3.

59. "Decision of the CCP Central Committee, the State Council, The Military Commission of the Central Committee and the Cultural Revolution Group Under the Central Committee Concerning the Resolute Support of People's Liberation Army for the Revolutionary Masses of the Left," CCP Documents of the Great Proletarian Cultural Revolution 1966-1967, p. 196.

60. Ch'üan-wu-ti [Invincible], no. 6, p. 3.

61. See Appendix C for names of Red Rebel and Red Guard organizations; see also, Ch'üan-wu-ti [Invincible], no. 6, p. 3.

62. Ch'üan-wu-ti [Invincible], no. 6, p. 3.

63. Ch'üan-wu-ti [Invincible], no. 6, p. 3.

64. Ch'üan-wu-ti [Invincible], no. 9.

65. "Order of the Central Military Commission," CCP Documents of the Great Proletarian Cultural Revolution 1966-1967, p. 409.

66. Ch'üan-wu-ti [Invincible], no. 9, translated in SCMP-S, no. 204.

67. Ch'üan-wu-ti [Invincible], no. 13, p. 1.

68. Robinson, "Chou En-lai and the Cultural Revolution in China," p. 215; see also, Klein, "The State Council and the Cultural Revolution," pp. 351-372.

69. David M. Lampton, Interview File 21 E, no. 6.

70. David M. Lampton, Interview File 21 E; see also, Who's Who in Communist China, p. 158.

71. David M. Lampton, Interview File 21 E, nos. 4 and 6.

72. David M. Lampton, "Trends in Health Policy," Current Scene 12, no. 6 (1974):5-6.

Chapter 10
POLICY CHANGE AND THE
AGENDA FOR THE
FUTURE (1968-1977)

<u>INTRODUCTION</u>

While the purposes and interests which were
served during the Great Proletarian Cultural Revolution were as diverse as the groups that participated
in the movement, medical policies did change in 1968.
This chapter will examine those alternations in the
policy areas where change was most conspicuous:
medical education, health service delivery, and
health financing. After having examined these policies, we shall specify their long and short-term
consequences. Finally, we shall look at the forces
that have brought about the reappearance of pre-
Cultural Revolution medical leadership in the 1973-
1977 period.

By 1968, the Ministry of Public Health appears
to have become largely irrelevant to the formulation
of the major contours of medical policy. All of the
<u>Wei-sheng-pu</u>'s principal pre-Cultural Revolution
leaders had been purged, army representatives with
little or no medical experience had titular control,
and major organizations such as hospitals and medical schools were torn by factionalism. Not only did
these problems virtually immobilize the Ministry and
make it ineffective as a participant in the policy-
making process, the power to make decisions across
a broad range of issues had been removed from the
bureaucracy and lodged with leaders at the Party
Center, the most conspicuous of which was Mao.[1]
This concentration of policy-making power had several consequences, but two were particularly important: First, because the number of matters competing
for the Chairman's attention was enormous, those
medical directives which were issued were few in
number, national in scope, and general. Secondly,
because central directives were not sufficiently
mediated and specified by the bureaucracy, local

leaders who were responsible for starting and nur-
turing these new programs faced enormous uncertainties. Delay and caution were the frequent result.

While this policy-making system had severe defects, as we shall see in the following chapter, it
did make it possible to achieve policy change and
coordination in the areas that were of the most concern to Mao: medical education, health delivery,
and rural financing.[2] Unlike the Great Leap Forward,
when the medical education system failed to change
in ways that were consistent with the alterations
being made in the health delivery system, some
degree of coordination was achieved in 1968. Such
coordination, however, was obtained at the considerable cost of creating local uncertainties, bureaucratic immobilization, and alienation of medical
professionals. These costs, along with the specific
defects of the policies, produced a trend toward the
reappearance of pre-Cultural Revolution medical
leadership in the 1973-1977 period. The central
issue of the 1970s has been, what have been the
costs and gains of the Cultural Revolution and how
much of its legacy should be preserved?

HEALTH POLICIES IN THE IMMEDIATE POST-CULTURAL
REVOLUTION PERIOD

Medical education at the higher level. In
March 1968, the Party Center issued guidelines on
medical education which reduced its length to a maximum of three years. "The period of schooling
should not be too long; we suggest that three years
is sufficient."[3] Because medical schools were so
faction-ridden, it was 1969-1970 before classes
could meet. The length of medical education, at
first, tended to be shorter than three years, only
achieving the proposed figure in 1971-1972.[4] One
presumes that educational authorities felt it was
preferable to err on the "radical" side. Between
the political uncertainties confronting medical
school administrators, and their uncertainty about
what a greatly shortened curriculum could usefully
look like, the medical schools faced a long period
of immobilization.

Concurrent with curricula reforms, there were
changes in admissions policies. "Graduates from
primary school and from junior middle school should
be admitted." This 1968 directive went on to say,

A part of the personnel and material resources
left in the cities should be utilized to open

227

advanced courses which admit as students those medical workers who have worked at the grass-roots level for several years and who are sound ideologically and need further technical training. . . . No limits regarding the period of schooling and the age of students should be placed.[5]

A Red Flag article in November amplified, saying that medical schools should primarily enroll "bare-foot doctors" (ch'ih-chiao i-sheng).[6] The final area of higher medical education policy to change was the location of medical training.

. . . medical units and prevention units in the cities should gradually move to the countryside. In this way, a large number of doctors can be trained within a short period of time to meet the needs of the broad masses. . . .[7]

For instance, Canton City's Chungshan (Sun Yat-sen) Medical School moved a portion of its facilities to rural areas, as did Shengyang Medical College.[8] Just how dramatically such changes actually redistributed educational resources and changed patterns of student admission is uncertain without comprehensive national data. However, my 1976 visit to Chungshan Medical School began to shed some light on this question. In 1970, Chungshan established a fifty-bed hospital in an outlying county which was supposed to train rural medical personnel, especially barefoot doctors;[9] it emphasized traditional medicine in its curriculum. This hospital, however, must be viewed against the fact that the Chungshan medical complex in Canton consists of five affiliated hospitals, one of which has 700 beds. In short, while medical schools were called upon to decentralize their training, the focus of activity for the major facilities appears to have remained in the cities.

Paramedic training. In October 1968, the "barefoot doctor" program, which had been first developed near Shanghai in 1958, was resurrected and promoted as national policy. Barefoot doctors were to be trained in regular classes at either the county or the commune hospital, or they were to be instructed by mobile medical teams coming from either the county or the commune.[10] Which method and level was to be utilized in any particular locality depended on the relative prosperity, size, distance, and capacity of the units concerned. The length of training was not specified, but three to six months encompasses the range of variation.

Selection of paramedic personnel was innovative with the local community having the responsibility to decide who would receive medical training. Because of the emphasis on vertical mobility among paraprofessionals, the new policy was theoretically giving the community an important voice in determining the future composition of the medical profession.

Implementation of these policies was relatively rapid because county hospitals were functioning normally before medical schools. In addition, because the Cultural Revolution had been much less disruptive in rural areas, extreme factionalism did not obstruct everything. Some provinces, however, were able to implement these plans more rapidly than others, with mismanagement, drought, dearth of funds, and lack of popular support obstructing the process in many provinces.[11] For instance, in 1971, only 50 percent of Shantung's production brigades had barefoot doctors while 85 percent of Shansi's brigades had such personnel.[12]

There appear to have been two reasons for the renewed emphasis on paramedics: First, the Cultural Revolution demonstrated that large sectors of the population had unmet health needs. Ways had to be found to keep central expenditures to a minimum while simultaneously making a dramatic effort to meet those needs. One way to do this was to siphon off manpower from counties to train rural personnel who would not be "divorced from agricultural production" and who could reduce the number of "unnecessary" referrals to higher levels. This policy has had costs, as we shall see. County hospitals have found their staffs further strained, hospital patients have had to wait longer, and some peasants have resented what they perceived was inferior rural care.[13] This emphasis on paramedics and a penetrating referral chain is consistent with both the pre-liberation medical legacy of the base areas and sound medical management. Despite the problems of such a system (and there are many), a paramedic based health system is the most efficient way to conserve scarce medical manpower, minimize costs, and provide timely treatment to a dispersed population. Subsequent analysis of China's difficulties in implementing this program should be viewed in this light.

Secondly, the training of barefoot doctors was a response to higher rural incomes.[14] The economic expansion of the mid-1960s created a situation in which it was possible for peasants to imagine allocating a small portion of their income to health care. This had not been the case during the serious economic decline of the early 1960s. The relationship between agricultural prosperity and the success of the barefoot doctor program is intimate. As data to be presented clearly demonstrate, the capacity to provide these services was (and is) directly tied to grain output.[15] When rural incomes decline, the pressure for cutting these programs increases.

<u>Policy vis à vis the structure of the health delivery system</u>. Because medical curricula should be designed with a specific delivery system in mind, a "rational" policy process would do that. While this had not occurred during the Great Leap Forward, it did in 1968. The rural health delivery system was modified in ways consonant with alterations being made in medical training. The "new" rural health programs initiated in the 1968-1969 period drew heavily upon previous experiments, taking account of some of the difficulties which had undermined those earlier efforts. The crisis experiments of 1960 and 1961 were most relevant because an attempt had been made to maintain collective ownership of health facilities and, at the same time, reduce production disincentives and excessive utilization of medical facilities.

While implementation of the new delivery policies was uneven, the objective was to have a comprehensive hospital in every district, a health office or hospital in every commune, barefoot doctors in each production brigade, and "health personnel" in every production team. The county hospital was responsible for training the rural medical personnel and for being the major referral facility when critical cases arose.[16] The commune clinic was charged with providing major medical and surgical procedures, as well as extensive outpatient services.[17]

The lowest level in the curative system was to be the production brigade (approximately a village), each of which was supposed to have at least two "barefoot doctors." Each of these paramedics was responsible for undertaking preventive health measures, weeding out "frivolous" cases, treating those individuals with diseases with which he or she was competent to deal, and referring the remaining patients to commune facilities. The hope was that this system would not lead to the imposition of excessive burdens on either commune or county hospitals.

　　　. . . someone raised this question: "What should be done about the shortage of doctors

230

after the introduction of the cooperative medical service when the number of patients visiting the commune's clinics increases?"[18]

Of course, the capacity of barefoot doctors to play this role is directly related to the confidence patients have in them. This has been a continual problem; calls for better training have been constantly heard.[19]

Without more detailed information on the process by which medical policies were formulated during the 1968-1969 period, one can only speculate about the considerations and pressures which gave form to these policies. We do know, however, that county hospitals had faced chronic financial difficulties and that this system was designed to reduce, or at least control, patient loads at this level. In addition, if health care was to be provided the rural populace, then the bulk of the financial burden had to be placed on ruralites themselves while, at the same time, not creating severe agricultural disincentives. In short, policy-makers were responding to the medical needs of the peasantry while simultaneously trying to meet the financial and productive constraints which confronted them.

Cultural Revolution financial policy took a page out of the 1960 chapter. At that time, Vice-Minister of Public Health Hsu Yun-pei had proposed a financing scheme designed to maintain cooperative ownership of health facilities while, at the same time, reducing excessive utilization and collective economic burdens. In 1960 Hsu had said,

> At present, the ideal medical care system for commune members . . . is collective medical care. Under this system, the expenses for medical care are jointly shouldered by the individual members and the commune, and the funds are pooled collectively.[20]

While this proposal had proven unworkable in the economic circumstances of 1960-1961, in 1968 this plan looked workable. "A voluntary system run on the principle of mutual aid. Commune members pay a small fee every year. This plus funds from the commune make the cooperative medical fund. Treatment requires only a tiny registration fee and medicines are free."[21] Basically, "cooperative health care" (ho-tso chih-liao) is subsidized insurance, with limited (and variable) benefits for those requiring referral to higher-level hospitals. The vision of

231

free high quality rural health care was (and is) distant.

There were at least three variants of this program. People's Daily concisely explained each:[22] (1) The production brigade could be the unit of accounting; this had the drawback of not being able to provide comprehensive services and it covered a rather small population. (2) Several contiguous production brigades could form a consolidated fund. This would expand the range of services and make it possible for small units to establish programs. (3) Communes could be the units of insurance, with brigades making specified contributions. This had the advantage of expanding the insured base and making relatively extensive services conceivable. However, one principle is important; the larger the unit of insurance, the more difficult it is to control costs. While no precise figures were released concerning the prevalence of each type of plan, one news article asserted that about 70 percent of China's production brigades had implemented plan one.[23]

The general adoption of this pattern indicates that most brigade and commune leaders opted for a plan with relatively narrow geographical coverage, a plan which was less stable under severe economic conditions, and one which was less capable of supporting major medical work. The rationale? It made it easier to control waste and overutilization and it minimized the subsidization of poorer units which well-to-do units resist. As one commune cadre noted,

. . . it is better to put cooperative medical funds under the central control of production brigades, so that they can keep their hands on such money and ideological work. Apart from this, the expenditure of too much money on some patients also affects the consolidation of the cooperative medical service.[24]

Because of these efforts to control costs, catastrophic illness can still impose backbreaking burdens. How frequently this has happened is simply unknown.

For instance, medical expenses in excess of 100 [yüan] ¥ are to be covered by individual patients through consultations with the production teams and on the basis of the financial conditions of the patients concerned. In such cases, the excess portions may either be

232

reduced cr exempted after they are discussed by poor and lower-middle peasants.[25]

One would anticipate that local willingness to cover an individual's bills would be a function of local prosperity and the class standing of the individual. The better the year, the more prosperous the unit, and the poorer the individual, the more likely it was (and is) that catastrophic costs would be covered.

Financing urban services is a subject which need not detain us; the Cultural Revolution had little apparent impact. For a brief period in 1967, some workers had been able to force their way into medical facilities, but the People's Liberation Army quickly ended that practice.[26] Once again (1977), there are contract, temporary, and part-time laborers who receive virtually none of the benefits extended regular heavy industrial workers and all government and Party personnel.[27] The effect of this inertia on the morale of those persons who were mobilized to attack the Wei-sheng-pu can only be surmised, but the lack of movement is testimony to the fact that leadership is constrained by objective factors which are not highly manipulatable.[28]

Pharmaceutical prices have a great impact on the solvency of cooperative health programs and are important in determining the quality of care available to all but those of elite status. Those agencies and individuals responsible for fixing drug prices had to decide whether it was preferable to keep price up, and reduce demand, or to increase availability at the possible short-run expense of quality or at the risk of creating shortages. In the mid-1960s, Po I-po and the pharmaceutical trust had pursued the strategy of fixing relatively higher prices and ensuring quality. With the "elimination" of the drug trust, prices declined an average of 37 percent in 1969.[29]

Not knowing which drugs were reduced how much, it is impossible to evaluate the impact of this move. The way in which the leadership sought to minimize the impact of the price reduction on demand was to encourage conservation of drugs (which was not terribly effective in the past) and to promote the use of traditional pharmaceuticals.[30] Several factors are important in determining the success of this approach: (a) How rapidly will pharmaceutical output grow? This is largely dependent on the rate of investment in the pharmaceutical industry. (b) Will the populace use traditional pharmaceuticals in

233

sufficient quantities to reduce the demand for "modern" drugs? (c) Will peasants be willing to devote scarce land to growing traditional medicinals? The answer to this depends upon agricultural well-being and alternative uses of the land. (d) Finally, are doctors and administrators sufficiently secure to resist wasteful demands for drugs?

Policy in the remaining issue areas. The financial, educational and delivery policies discussed above were formulated in 1968 at levels well above the Wei-sheng-pu, although it is not clear who the most salient policy-makers were. This type of "centrally-coordinated" policy-making system had several advantages, the most important of which was its capacity to achieve policy coherence. Unlike the Great Leap Forward, educational, financial, and structural decisions were made in the same arena using the same assumptions. Consequently, all three areas of policy reinforced one another.

While the next chapter will analyze this system in greater detail, one major problem was that relatively few areas of policy received attention. The emergence of policy was slower in those issue areas which were peripheral to immediate concerns. As a consequence, policy vis à vis medical research, mass campaigns, Chung-i, and the conditions of physician employment were slow in being formulated. Only with the gradual reemergence of the Ministry as a vigorous policy-maker in the 1970s have these important areas received attention. Quite predictably, as the site of decision-making has moved back to the Ministry in the 1973-1977 period, policy has increasingly reflected the perceptions and goals of those sectors of Chinese society with access to that political arena.

POLICY PROBLEMS AND LEADERSHIP CHANGE IN THE POST-CULTURAL REVOLUTION ERA

By the first years of the 1970s, several serious, and possibly unanticipated, consequences of Cultural Revolution medical policy became apparent. These obstacles have provided the momentum for both policy and leadership change in the 1973-1977 period. These problems, changes, and turmoil have had their equivalents in other policy areas such as: education, foreign relations, agriculture, and industrial management, just to mention a few. The debate over how much of the Cultural Revolution legacy should be preserved certainly has not been confined to

234

medicine, as the October 1976 purge of the "gang of four" (ssu jen pang) has amply demonstrated.[31]

Medical education policy confronted two diffi- culties in its immediate post-Cultural Revolution form: First, the concept of a referral chain in which county and commune health centers play major curative roles requires that the physicians at these levels possess relatively broad medical skills. Additionally, the specialty hospitals at higher levels of the referral chain require specialists with substantial training, informal or otherwise. The problem which medical educators have faced is simply producing omnicompetent individuals in three years while, at the same time, meeting the system's requirements for specialists. The arduous nature of this task was evident in the fact that most medical schools debated for two to three years how to con- struct an abbreviated curriculum.[32]

The difficulties in implementing such a course of instruction were compounded by two additional considerations: (1) Because of the political cri- teria which governed medical school admission, stu- dents frequently lacked adequate preparation, prepar- ation which was especially important given the accelerated curriculum. (2) Whereas medical schools in other countries can depend on enrolling students with substantial premedical education (obtained in secondary or higher schools), Chinese medical schools could not take such preparation for granted, until possibly recently.[33] In short, medical schools were asked to take more poorly prepared students, train them to be omnicompetent physicians, and do all of this in one-half the time consumed prior to the Cultural Revolution. Also, Cultural Revolution medical education policy made no specific provisions for specialty training, a particularly critical omission, considering the importance of such indi- viduals in a referral chain.

Given these difficulties, medical educators and some Wei-sheng-pu officials have pushed as delicate- ly as possible for alterations in policy. These efforts have had visible impact in the 1973-1977 period, though the precise mechanism by which such influence has been exercised remains obscure. While it is unwarranted to draw major conclusions from one interviewee, one medical doctor (1972) expressed a view that seemed to presage recent changes in the educational sphere.

. . . there ought to be many doctors with les- ser education than that [three years], and lots

235

with more; . . . total reliance on partially
trained persons is particularly dangerous. . . .
Most doctors agree with this. . . . Three years
were not enough because most of the students
have no scientific background that a medical
school in the West would take for granted.

I then asked this interviewee how curriculum revi-
sions would occur.

. . . as long as Mao is alive there will be no
formal changes but there will be informal
changes. . . . One way . . . is to have students, upon graduation from three-year medical
school, engage in advanced study or to have
higher degrees of middle school preparation.[34]

Indeed, the changes which this respondent pre-
dicted were not long in coming. In 1973, Chungshan
Medical School in Canton lengthened its curriculum
by six months, with the addition of a "fundamental
course."[35] Along with alterations in curriculum,
1973 also witnessed a renewed emphasis on written
and oral examinations.[36] The dissatisfactions with,
and changes in, medical education were indicative of
a generalized dissatisfaction with the entire post-
Cultural Revolution educational system. By the
second half of 1975, then Minister of Education Chou
Jung-hsin, and Liu Ping, the vice-president of
Tsinghua University, called for comprehensive alterations in all educational programs. In August and
October 1975, Liu and two colleagues wrote Chairman
Mao Tse-tung a letter in which they are alleged to
have said that students graduating from the post-
Cultural Revolution system were "not even capable of
reading a book. . . ."[37] At about the same time,
Liu is reputed to have asserted that, ". . . students graduating from universities were unable to
recognize the letters A.B.C.D." and that "schools
open to all are leftwing."[38] While one must be
careful in writing either political or policy obitu-
aries in China, the September 9, 1976 death of Mao,
and the subsequent purge of the "gang of four,"
would seem to have removed many of the impediments
to major changes in the educational sphere.[39]
    Dissatisfaction with post-Cultural Revolution
medical education has not been confined to the
"regular" medical school curriculum. Methods of
instructing barefoot doctors have come in for criticism. The level and quality of training which barefoot doctors receive is an important determinant of

the success of the entire rural medical program. If
peasants do not have faith in the capacities of
these paramedics they demand referral to higher (and
more expensive) facilities, thereby increasing the
burdens of such institutions.

> . . . the inexperience of the "barefoot doctors"
> and the shortage of good medicine are the main
> reasons why city hospitals are over-crowded
> with patients from rural areas seeking treat-
> ment. . . .[40]

In the 1972-1974 period, the press frequently
printed denunciations of individuals who claimed
that barefoot doctors were inadequately trained and,
in some cases, incompetent.[41] While denouncing
those who criticized barefoot doctors, the regime
took their criticisms seriously and modified policy.
Increasing emphasis has been placed on quality education for barefoot doctors, in particular longer
training. By mid-1976, Fengchen County, Inner Mongolia, was being praised for having established a
barefoot doctor program of one and one-half years
duration.[42] In the wake of the 1976 purge of the
"gang of four," many provinces convened conferences
devoted to improving the barefoot doctor program.[43]
Health care delivery policy was one of the major
foci of Cultural Revolution change. Most conspicuous was the emphasis placed upon rural areas and the
promotion of the cooperative health program. While
there is little indication that anyone in China has
seriously proposed wholesale abandonment of these
emphases and programs, rural and urban health care
have encountered obstacles, and remedial actions
have been debated and implemented. Change has become increasingly pronounced in the 1973-1977 period.
Two difficulties have been of overriding importance: First, because cooperative health programs
are supported by a combination of collective funds
(which receive a fixed percentage of local rural
production) and individual peasant contributions,
the capacity to provide these services is directly
tied to the productivity and stability of the local
economic base. Secondly, because of the increased
availability of rural curative services, commune and
county institutions have frequently been overburdened and cooperative health programs bankrupted by
the expense of referral and treatment.
The most severe problem facing the cooperative
health system has been its high degree of dependence
upon local agricultural production. In 1972, China's

237

grain output declined approximately 4 percent.[44]
Shortly thereafter, the mass media carried numerous
denunciations of cadres who terminated cooperative
health programs for allegedly economic reasons.
For instance, in August 1972, the leadership of one
production brigade in Shihpaliku Commune, Hsin
County, Shantung Province, terminated its health
program because the brigade ". . . could no longer
afford the medical cooperative system . . ." and
because ". . . economic conditions were so poor here
and commune members had no money. . . ."[45]

The relationship between local economic well-
being and program viability holds not only for selec-
tive qualitative data, it also is evident in the
imperfect aggregate national data we have. For
example, in 1972 Kwangtung experienced a drop in
grain output; the following year that province
reported a decline in the percentage of its production brigades with cooperative health programs. In
1975, Kwangtung once again suffered a grain output
decline and, once again, the following year brought
a reduction in the percentage of production brigades
providing cooperative services.[46] Conversely, in
ten of the thirteen instances in which we have the
necessary information, ". . . provincial foodgrain
increases one year were followed the next by increases in the availability of cooperative health
programs within these same provinces. . . ."[47] Concisely, it has been difficult to assure program continuity in the absence of agricultural stability.

Cooperative health programs have faced difficulty from another quarter as well; excessive demand
for services, high rates of referral to commune and
county facilities (to which payments must then be
made), and requests for relatively expensive pharmaceuticals. As one article candidly noted,

> There were also some commune members who
> thought that they could make something out of
> this. Regardless of whether they were seri-
> ously ill or slightly indisposed, they went to
> [the] hospital to see the doctor regularly and
> asked for good medicine. More money was thus
> spent, and the doctors also were kept busy all
> the time.[48]

Red Flag noted that,

> The funds for running the cooperative medical
> stations are limited. Therefore, it is neces-
> sary to run them diligently and frugally. Some

of the cooperative medical stations are unaware
of this point and spend money freely . . . As
a result, funds are quickly exhausted and the
cooperative medical services are unable to
continue operating.[49]

As a consequence of these assorted problems,
one particularly significant policy initiative was
taken in order to enhance the solvency of these programs. In 1973, the regime announced that it was
subsidizing at least some cooperative health services.[50] Money was being provided to cover both
operating and capital costs. This is, of course, a
risky path for the central government to pursue.
Subsidies in China, as elsewhere, tend to breed
dependence and larger requests for funds. It is
unknown how widespread direct subsidization has
become, however, during the first half of the 1970s
increasingly large portions of provincial health
budgets were being expended in rural areas.[51]
As explained in two previous chapters, the
cooperative health system was seen by Mao as a means
by which to increase the emphasis on rural areas.
Prior to the Cultural Revolution, urban politicians
such as P'eng Chen, hospital administrators, and the
Wei-sheng-pu had resisted rapid diffusion of resources partly out of fear that this would precipi-
tate a deterioration in city services. While there
are virtually no data which document a decline in
urban services, the 1976 purge of the "gang of four"
has brought hints that this may have occurred.
Equally important, the purge has brought demands
that selected social groups receive added attention,
particularly cadres.
In the early and mid-1960s, Ministry of Public
Health leaders such as Ch'ien Hsin-chung and urbanites like P'eng Chen stressed the need to give equal
emphasis to city and countryside. During the Cultural Revolution and its aftermath, this formula was
rejected in favor of Mao's June 1965 slogan, "In
medical and health work place the stress on the
rural areas" (pa i-liao wei-sheng te chung-tien fang
tao nung-ts'un ch'ü ma).[52] The pre-Cultural Revolution formula is, once again, being articulated.
From December 12-20, 1976, provincial authorities
in Szechwan convened a barefoot doctors conference
at which it was resolved to treat urban and rural
areas more equally. This meeting denounced the
"gang of four" for having opposed the following
policy.

We wanted to place stress on the rural areas in
medical and public health work and, while
strengthening the building of rural public
health work, grasp well public health work in
factories and mines and in cities.[53]

In the same way that the Cultural Revolution
had attacked the prior urban bias of the health system, cadre privilege had come under attack. While
no available information documents that there was an
actual reduction in cadre privilege vis à vis medical care in the 1968-1975 period, Party members are
now asserting that they were discriminated against
in the post-Cultural Revolution period. Formerly
privileged groups now seem to be claiming that the
Cultural Revolution brought a real reduction in the
quality, or at least availability, of care for them.
For instance, in January 1977, public health workers
and Party cadres in Shanghai said that,

> . . . medical treatment was denied to many
> leading cadres in Shanghai by the "gang of
> four." A veteran Red Army cadre . . . became
> an outpatient because hospitalization was no
> longer available to him. Wang Hung-wen and
> Chang Ch'un-ch'iao [two members of the "gang
> of four"] even went so far as to personally
> order some hospitals to discharge certain num-
> bers of responsible comrades from other provin-
> ces and cities. All this shows that the "gang
> of four" utilized the major power in the field
> of medical and health work to attack and delib-
> erately harass the leading revolutionary
> cadres. . . .[54]

What seems to be occurring [1977] is the reemergence of a coalition that was important prior to the
Cultural Revolution. Party cadres, city administrators, and much of the medical community all have a
common interest in adequate levels of urban care.
They appear to have acquired sufficient security to
articulate those interests once again. How far this
retrenchment should proceed is undoubtedly being
debated in Peking.

ACCOMPANYING LEADERSHIP CHANGE

As documented throughout this study, leadership
change frequently accompanies policy alterations.
This observation leaves open the question of whether

240

such changes produce those shifts or merely reflect them. I have concluded that leadership change both reflects fundamental resource and political alterations and lends additional momentum to them. Leadership plays an important role in defining the problems to which the system addresses itself. Since 1973, a striking restoration of pre-Cultural Revolution Ministry of Public Health leadership has taken place. In fact, Cultural Revolution casualties have reemerged in great numbers in all areas and levels of the society. It has been this clash between the victims of the Cultural Revolution and its chief beneficiaries that has provided the dynamic to Chinese politics in the 1970s.

The first Ministry of Public Health resurrection of a Cultural Revolution casualty occurred in late 1973 when it was announced that former Minister Ch'ien Hsin-chung was "a leading member" of the Wei-sheng-pu.[55] Ch'ien had long been associated with an emphasis on research and thorough medical education. His reappearance coincided with the resumption of publication of the Chinese Medical Journal. Ch'ien's resurrection seems to have signalled the regime's recognition of the policy problems identified above, especially those relating to medical education and research. Shortly after Ch'ien reappeared, the former director of the Health Services Bureau, Huang Shu-tse, was revived politically. He assumed a vice-ministerial post in the Wei-sheng-pu.[56] During the Cultural Revolution, both Ch'ien and Huang had been major targets of Red Rebel and Red Guard attack for their alleged devotion to urban focused and elite oriented medical care.

Significantly, two additional personnel changes have solidified the trend toward the dominance of the pre-Cultural Revolution leadership. In 1973 Dr. Huang Chia-ssu, the pre-1966 head of the Chinese Academy of Medical Sciences, and a strong counterweight to Mao's 1965 views on medical education, had reemerged as the head of that organization.[57] Equally important, Ch'ien's post-Cultural Revolution successor as minister of public health, Liu Hsiang-p'ing (the widow of Hsieh Fu-chih), is now being denounced as the representative of the "gang of four" in the Ministry.[58]

While there is an enormous amount that remains unknown about the present composition and predispositions of China's health policy-makers,[59] it is clear that the late 1970s are likely to witness an increasingly open critique of Cultural Revolution medical policy. However, it is highly unlikely that this reevaluation will lead to a wholesale dismemberment of all Cultural Revolution health programs. This is so simply because China's peasantry has now come to expect health care, the Ministry of Public Health is committed to providing it, and a mass-oriented paramedic system is the only way to do so, given the resource constraints and the enormity of the population involved. Within these limits, though, the future will likely see more emphasis placed on research and "quality" medical education. The precise balance to be achieved between immediate health needs and future growth and development will be the subject of as much debate in the next twenty-eight years as it has been during the last twenty-eight.

ON COSTS AND GAINS

Tentatively evaluating the costs and gains of the Cultural Revolution in health is not the same as asking, "Was the entire movement worth it?" To answer the latter query would require a full assessment of losses and gains across all areas of policy. These gains and losses may not be fully apparent for years to come, if ever. Even more fundamentally, the weight one assigns to various losses and gains is, of course, a function of the values one holds. Finally, one would have to specify where pre-Cultural Revolution policy would have led had there been no movement at all, an almost metaphysical task. Consequently, I will merely identify the immediately apparent costs and gains of the movement, leaving the question of "Was it worth it?" to future analysts.

(1) The first important cost was an aggravation of a difficulty which all socialist countries have. There is no legitimate means by which to allocate scarce health services; medical care is a human right. This desire to make medical care universally available on an equitable and inexpensive basis has come into conflict with an overwhelming reality; medicine, doctors, instruments, and facilities are scarce and allocation must occur through either formal or informal mechanisms. In China, both formal and informal guidelines have been used, and both have created hostility among those who were not the beneficiaries. While Mao could effectively mobilize people over this issue, and temporarily change the policy-makers, he could not eliminate the need for allocation itself. This being the case, the Chairman seems to have raised hopes that could not be

met, at least immediately. In the process, he may have both placed bureaucrats in an untenable position and raised the general level of frustration.

(2) Doctors are virtually the only people who can control hospital waste and overutilization. Professional oversight is absolutely essential if medical facilities are to serve the most people in the most economical fashion. The exercise of such control, however, implies that doctors will tell cadres, workers, and others that they do not need specific care. Yet, during the Cultural Revolution, it was precisely workers, cadres, and government employees who most vehemently attacked doctors for their "callousness." In short, the Cultural Revolution decreased the physician's ability to say NO!

(3) Another cost was that an unknown number of highly trained physicians left the People's Republic in the post-Cultural Revolution period.[60] Most of these individuals were highly trained overseas Chinese who had come to China in the early 1960s. Their departure reduced China's immediate clinical, and long-term training, capabilities. A related cost was the fact that from 1967-1969, virtually all specialists were serving in outpatient clinics, or on mobile medical teams, where their advanced training was of minimal use. While there may have been ideological gains from such a policy, there were also major opportunity costs.

(4) During the four years that most medical schools were not operating, possibly in excess of 100,000 fully trained and intermediate-level doctors could have been produced; none were. In the future, there will be a period when doctors are retiring and there will be no equivalent skill pool to draw upon. Additionally, with schools only training three-year doctors, where will adequate numbers of experienced specialists come from?

Looking at the big picture, one ought to note that important gains have been made as well. It is clear that many more peasants have access to some level of health care than ever before and that financial resources are being distributed more evenly. The movement reemphasized the concept of equality, even if its immediate realization is difficult to achieve. Equally important, Cultural Revolution health policy came to terms with a problem all medical systems face. How can medical care be provided to everyone if it is delivered exclusively in a capital intensive and highly technical environment by only highly trained professionals? The creation of a broad spectrum of health personnel

243

is essential in order to provide timely, economical, and convenient care to patients while keeping system costs manageable. This is especially true in an agricultural society. When all is said and done, this general concept will outlast the specific provisions of Cultural Revolution medical policy. How one weighs these gains against the costs outlined above is a question of values and will be a driving force in health politics for years to come.

SUMMARY

The immediate result of the Cultural Revolution was to create a "centrally-coordinated" system in which educational, financial, and delivery policies were aimed at solving fundamental health problems in the rural areas. Because of the limited time and knowledge of central leaders, as well as their priorities, some policy areas (e.g., medical research) were neglected. With the increasingly prominent role of the Ministry of Public Health in the 1970s, there have been changes in aspects of Cultural Revolution education and financial policy, and guidelines for medical research and professional life have appeared. These changes have reflected an increased level of professional influence in the policy-making process. The "new" leadership to emerge in the 1973-1977 period appears to be characterized by individuals (such as Ch'ien Hsin-chung) who have a long public record of favoring research, exhaustive medical training, and quality care. While it would be a mistake to attribute a set of values to leaders simply because they are medical professionals, the new leaders have already begun to initiate policies which are consistent with their past positions and background.

While Cultural Revolution medical policy will undoubtedly undergo change, the status quo ante is unlikely to be restored. A corps of medical workers has been created, a referral chain now exists, and China's peasants have had their demands for medical care legitimated. This represents a monumental achievement.

NOTES

1. Analysts of Chinese politics during this period know very little about either the mechanisms by which decisions were made or the personalities that

played decisive roles, especially in specific policy areas.

2.   Mao's concern with these dimensions of medical policy was clearly demonstrated in his June 26, 1965 "Directive on Medical Work." See, Mao Tse-tung, "Tui Wei-sheng Kung-tso Te Chih-shih" [Directive on medical work], in Mao Tse-tung Ssu-hsiang Wan-sui [Long live the thought of Mao Tse-tung] (Peking: 1969), pp. 615-616.

3.   "Medical Education Must be Transformed on the Basis of Mao Tse-tung's Thought," China's Medicine 3 (1968):163.

4.   Roland Berger, "Medical Training in China," Eastern Horizon 12, no. 1 (1973):31-34.

5.   "Medical Education Must be Transformed on the Basis of Mao Tse-tung's Thought," p. 163.

6.   "The Orientation of the Revolution in Medical Education as Seen in the Growth of Barefoot Doctors," Hung Ch'i [Red flag], no. 3 (1968), cited in China's Medicine 10 (1968):574-581.

7.   "Medical Education Must Be Transformed on the Basis of Mao Tse-tung's Thought," p. 163.

8.   "After the Period of Schooling was Shortened," China Reconstructs 20, no. 11 (1971):17-19.

9.   David M. Lampton, Trip Notes (October 1976).

10.   "The Orientation of the Revolution in Medical Education as Seen in the Growth of Barefoot Doctors."

11.   Chin Wei, "Continue to Carry Out Well the Revolution in Public Health in the Countryside," Red Flag, no. 12 (1973), in Foreign Broadcast Information Service, Daily Report: People's Republic of China (hereafter FBIS), no. 245 (1973), pp. B 3-B 9.

12.   David M. Lampton, "The Roots of Inequality in Education and Health Services in China: A First Look at Five Provinces" (Presented at the Thirtieth International Congress of Human Sciences in Asia and North Africa, Mexico City, Mexico, August 3-8, 1976), p. 43.

13.   Ta-chung Jih-pao [The masses daily], March 20,

1974, Tsinan Provincial Service in Mandarin, March 20, 1974, in FBIS, no. 61 (1974), pp. C 1-C 4.

14. While we know very little about real income levels in rural areas, Eckstein and Orleans assert that per capita gross national product rose from a base of 100 in 1952 to 148.5 in 1959 and then fell to 119.6 in 1963. By 1966, it had climbed to 147.1 and was 177.2 in 1970. See Alexander Eckstein, "Economic Growth and Change in China: A Twenty-Year Perspective," China Quarterly, no. 54 (1973), p. 232.

15. David M. Lampton, "Economics, Politics, and the Determinants of Policy Outcomes in China: Post-Cultural Revolution Health Policy," The Australian and New Zealand Journal of Sociology 12, no. 1 (1976): 43-49.

16. "An Investigation Report on How the Ch'ünhsing Brigade in Ch'üchiang Hsien, Kwangtung Province Firmly Adheres to Cooperative Medical Service Over the Past Eleven Years," Hung Ch'i [Red flag], no. 1 (1969), in Survey of China Mainland Magazines (hereafter SCMM), no. 642.

17. "A Good Thing Since Creation," Jen-min Jih-pao [People's daily], December 8, 1968, in Current Background (hereafter CB), no. 872, p. 11.

18. "Cooperative Medical Service is Just Fine," Jen-min Jih-pao [People's daily], December 8, 1968, CB, no. 872, p. 9.

19. Hangchow, Chekiang Provincial Service, February 27, 1974.

20. Hsu Yun-pei, "Advance the Great Work of Protecting the People's Health," Chinese Medical Journal 80 (1960):412-413.

21. "Everybody Works for Good Health," China Reconstructs 20, no. 11 (1971):21.

22. "A Great Revolution on the Health Front," Jen-min Jih-pao [People's daily], December 13, 1968, CB, no. 872, p. 14.

23. "Medical Care for 700 Million," China Reconstructs 21, no. 11 (1972):14-15.

24. "The Views of the Huangts'un and Lianghsiang Communes on the Cooperative Medical Service in Force

at the Loyüan Commune," <u>Jen-min Jih-pao</u> [People's daily], December 5, 1968, <u>CB</u>, no. 872, p. 5.

25. "Cooperative Medical Service is Just Fine," <u>Jen-min Jih-pao</u> [People's daily], December 8, 1968, <u>CB</u>, no. 872, p. 8.

26. David M. Lampton, <u>Interview File 21 E</u>.

27. For more on the stratification of workers see, Lynn T. White III, "Workers' Politics in Shanghai," <u>Journal of Asian Studies</u> 36, no. 1 (1976):99-116.

28. David M. Lampton, <u>Health, Conflict, and the Chinese Political System</u>, Michigan Papers in Chinese Studies, no. 18 (Ann Arbor: Center for Chinese Studies, 1974), Chapter 1.

29. "Big Nationwide Reduction of Medicine Prices," <u>New China News Agency</u> (hereafter <u>NCNA</u>), September 25, 1969, in <u>Survey of the China Mainland Press</u> (hereafter <u>SCMP</u>), no. 4508, p. 19.

30. "Rely on Mao Tse-tung's Thought to Uncover the Motherland's Great Treasures of Medicine," <u>Jen-min Jih-pao</u> [People's daily], March 1, 1969, in <u>SCMP</u>, no. 4375, pp. 6-11.

31. Mao's widow, Chiang Ch'ing, and three male allies from Shanghai (Wang Hung-wen, Yao Wen-yuan, and Chang Ch'un-ch'iao), collectively are known as the "gang of four." These four were closely identi-fied with Cultural Revolution excesses. The September 1976 death of Mao removed the major obstacle to their purge.

32. Roland Berger, "Medical Training in China," <u>Eastern Horizon</u> 12, no. 1 (1973):28-36.

33. E. Grey Dimond, "Medical School Curriculum in the People's Republic of China," <u>Journal of the American Medical Association</u> 236, no. 13 (1976): 1489-1491.

34. David M. Lampton, <u>Interview File 21 E</u>, no. 6, pp. 3-4.

35. David M. Lampton, "Trends in Health Policy," <u>Current Scene</u> 12, no. 6 (1974):6-7.

36. <u>Ta Kung Pao</u> [Impartial daily], November 16, 1973; see also, Lampton, "Trends in Health Policy,"

pp. 6-7; see also, Hofei, Anhwei Provincial Service in Mandarin, August 4, 1974, FBIS, no. 153 (1974), p. G 1.

37. Agence France Presse (hereafter AFP), December 9, 1975, in FBIS, no. 237 (1975), p. E 7.

38. AFP, December 24, 1975, in FBIS, no. 248 (1975), p. E 5.

39. In fact, Kuang-ming Jih-pao [Bright daily], December 12, 1976, attacked the "gang of four" for ". . . instilling fear in the minds of teachers who taught seriously and students who studied diligently." See FBIS, no. 252 (1976), p. E 10.

40. "Stepping-up the Services of Barefoot Doctors," South China Morning Post, February 1, 1973, p. 13; cited in, Lampton, "Trends in Health Policy," p. 3.

41. For instance see, Hangchow, Chekiang Provincial Service in Mandarin, February 27, 1974.

42. Huhehot, Inner Mongolia Regional Service in Mandarin, July 9, 1976, in FBIS, no. 134 (1976), p. K 3.

43. For instance, Szechwan Province held such a conference in December 1976. See, Ch'engtu, Szechwan Provincial Service in Mandarin, December 21, 1976, in FBIS, no. 248 (1976), pp. J 1-J 3.

44. Neville Maxwell, "Recent Chinese Grain Figures," China Quarterly, no. 68 (1976), p. 818.

45. Cited in Lampton, "Trends in Health Policy." p. 2.

46. Lampton, "The Roots of Inequality . . .," pp. 41-44.

47. Lampton, "The Roots of Inequality . . .," p. 40.

48. Jen-min Jih-pao [People's daily], December 19, 1968, in CB, no. 872, p. 18.

49. Chin Wei, p. 3.

50. "Co-op Medical Care in Sun Village," China Reconstructs 21, no. 11 (1972):6.

51. Lampton, "Trends in Health Policy," p. 4.

52. Mao Tse-tung, p. 616.

53. Ch'engtu, Szechwan Provincial Service in Mandarin, December 21, 1976, in FBIS, no. 248 (1976), p. J 2.

54. Shanghai City Service in Mandarin, January 12, 1977, in FBIS, no. 12 (1977), p. G 10.

55. NCNA, November 1, 1973, in FBIS, no. 212 (1973), p. A 13. On January 22, 1974, Ch'ien was said to be a vice-minister of public health. See, NCNA, January 22, 1974, in FBIS, no. 16 (1974), p. A 12.

56. NCNA, January 22, 1974, in FBIS, no. 16 (1974), p. A 12.

57. NCNA, July 8, 1976, in FBIS, no. 134 (1976), p. A 17.

58. AFP, January 10, 1977, in FBIS, no. 7 (1977), p. E 1; see also, AFP, December 1, 1976, in FBIS, no. 233 (1976), p. E 3.

59. For instance, we know virtually nothing about the background and predispositions of "leading persons" in the Wei-sheng-pu such as Chang Chih-chiang and Hsu Shou-jen. Also, we know little about Chu Chang-keng, vice-president of the Chinese Medical Association and Tu Pao-chang, deputy secretary-general of the Chinese Medical Association.

60. David M. Lampton, Interview File 21 E.

Chapter 11
PERSPECTIVE ON CHINESE POLICY-MAKING AND POLITICAL DEVELOPMENT (1949-1977)*

INTRODUCTION

The preceding chapters have intensively examined the political, economic and structural forces
which have generated health policies in China over
the last twenty-eight years. One thing has become
abundantly clear; leadership has been hemmed in from
all sides and compromise and conflict have frequently been the results. In these final pages we shall
move beyond the analysis of events and look at process, the process of political development and change
in the People's Republic as it appears from the vantage point of health care. The degree to which the
pattern of change observed in this issue area is gen-
eralizable is a matter for empirical investigation.
     The argument to be developed is that the last
twenty-eight years has witnessed a succession of
three types of health policy-making systems. By
systematically comparing these systems along the
following dimensions, we shall gain some understanding of the dynamics behind political change:
(1) How has authority been divided among the various
levels of the policy-making system? (2) Which interests have been accorded preferential access or
acquired "strategic positions" in the policy system?
(3) What kinds of information have dominated each
system and what impact has this had on leadership
perceptions? (4) How has each system encouraged or
inhibited coordination and innovation? (5) What are
the breakdowns to which each system is most vulnerable?

---

*An expanded version of this chapter appeared in,
David M. Lampton, Health, Conflict, and the Chinese
Political System, Papers in Chinese Studies, no. 18
(Ann Arbor: Center for Chinese Studies, 1974).

When Chairman Mao Tse-tung and his comrades came to power in 1949, the Chinese Communist Party was poorly equipped to handle the tidal wave of administrative demands with which it was deluged. This was especially true in the medical field where most of the doctors had been educated in foreign institutions, or by foreigners in Chinese schools. The Wei-sheng-pu was established in the context of massive tasks and limited manpower with a leadership composed largely of western-style medical doctors; all had had little identification with the Party's political apparatus. Below the vice-ministerial level, most bureau chiefs in substantive medical fields were medical doctors also. These individuals valued professional independence, consultation, and scientific medicine. In fact, this bundle of values brought the post-liberation Ministry into conflict with Party leaders, in particular Mao. This friction led to the reprimand of Tsui I-t'ien and the 1955-1956 purge of Wang Pin and Ho Ch'eng.

From an organizational perspective, this system was characterized by an hierarchically organized Ministry with relatively comprehensive policy-making authority. The Wei-sheng-pu was embedded in a bureaucratic context consisting of other ministries which had responsibilities which, to varying extents, overlapped its own. The central Party and state leadership assumed the role of referee by resolving disputes between ministries and setting broad programmatic objectives. Often this process occurred within the specialized systems (hsi-t'ung) of the central Party apparatus. This type of policy-making system will be called "bureaucratic" because it combined elements of central control with a broad range of ministerial independence. In fact, by 1955-1956, the independence and professional orientation of the Wei-sheng-pu had become the cause célèbre for the ouster of Dr. Ho Ch'eng, first vice-minister of public health.[1]

In response to the perceived independence of the Wei-sheng-pu, the increasing vitality of the central Party apparatus, and the alienation evident in the Hundred Flowers Campaign, the 1955-1958 period witnessed a transformation of the policy-making system. This occurred by progressively removing responsibilities from the Ministry and creating new arenas in which these issues could be handled. The first move was made in November 1955, with the establishment of the Nine Man Sub-committee on

251

Schistosomiasis.[2] By 1958, the Sub-committee's range of responsibilities had expanded to the point that it was responsible for all antiparasite work in China.[3] As noted, the Wei-sheng-pu resisted the diminution of its authority and resented the acquisition of clinical tasks by nonmedical personnel. Ministerial responsibilities declined not only with regard to parasitic diseases but also in the realm of rural health delivery. With the establishment of people's communes, these organizations assumed responsibility for curative health care below the county level.

From an administrative perspective, the bureaucratic system had been transformed into a "divided" policy-making system. Control of policy in a functionally unified area was fragmented among organizationally independent units. Coordinating policies being generated in several competing organizations proved to be difficult. This finally precipitated a reversion to the bureaucratic system in the 1960-1965 period.

The Cultural Revolution in health was a response to the characteristics of the bureaucratic system. When a new policy-making structure began to congeal out of the initial turbulence of the Cultural Revolution, it was extraordinarily dependent upon a small group of policy-makers at the pinnacles. While many observers have emphasized the delegation of authority away from ministries toward "revolutionary committees" in schools, factories, medical facilities, and communes, local authority was severely limited by the central directives dictating basic structural changes. For example, medical schools had leeway in devising three-year medical curricula; they did not have a role in deciding to have three-year curricula in the first place. Because basic policy authority was concentrated, the polity's lower participants were unable, or afraid, to take the initiative. This was a system that was critically dependent upon clear initiatives from the top.

The Ministry of Public Health, in the 1967-1969 period, was administrative in the narrowest sense of the word. One of the important consequences of this "centrally-coordinated" system was that new guidelines were slow in emerging.[4] The sluggishness of this system has been one of the major reasons for the movement toward a bureaucratic policy-making system in the post-1970 period.[5]

In short, the health policy-making system has tended toward a bureaucratic configuration in three periods: 1949-1955, 1960-1965, and 1970 to the present. There have been periodic attempts to move away from that structure; once in the 1955-1960 period, and once again in the 1967-1969 period. Each departure from this system was precipitated by specific system defects and each reappearance of the bureaucratic configuration was the result of even greater problems with the alternative structure.

The balance of this concluding chapter will outline the characteristics of each of these systems, define the instabilities of each, and develop a concept of political change and development in China. Having treated the bureaucratic system as an "equilibrium" form, we shall first describe the "divided" and "centrally-coordinated" configurations, saving the discussion of the "bureaucratic" system for the last.

DIVIDED POLICY-MAKING: ONE DIVIDES INTO TWO, 1955-1960

By late 1955, Chairman Mao asserted that the Ministry of Public Health was relatively more responsive to urban than rural curative health needs.[6] In response, the Nine Man Sub-committee on Schistosomiasis was established and placed under the direct supervision of the Party Central Committee. The Sub-committee was almost completely beyond Wei-sheng-pu influence. All known Sub-committee leaders were political personages with no medical experience. One had been involved in agricultural policy (Liao Lu-yen), two were political leaders in Shanghai (K'o Ch'ing-shih and Wei Wen-po), and one was a vice-minister of public health with no medical experience (Hsu Yun-pei). In short, the Sub-committee was an arena which embodied rural and political interests and objectives. This was a significantly different institution than the Ministry.

In August 1958, additional health responsibilities were given to organizations outside of the Ministry of Public Health, most important of which were the commune health centers under the control of local Party Committees. These new curative centers had little operational relationship to the Wei-sheng-pu and were charged with handling the bulk of clinical work below the county. The Commune Party Committees constituted an arena which embraced rural, political, and nonprofessional interests.

By August 1958, responsibilities for major health programs were lodged in three major institutional settings, each of which had little formal

253

relationship with the other. The Sub-committee and
the communes were entities in which nonprofessional
values, rural interests, and upwardly mobile (middle-
level) political cadres were dominant. In contrast,
the Wei-sheng-pu was responsible for major educational, research, and administrative programs and
was dominated by physicians who valued research,
"safety" in curative programs, and thorough training.
The leaders of the Sub-committee and the communes
were responsive to the Party political apparatus
while the Ministry high command had traditionally
been resistant to nonprofessional demands. With
three distinct political arenas operating in one
functional area, coordination became difficult.

The Sub-committee was a unique institution. Its
leadership was entirely nonmedical, with Party political cadres in charge.[7] Below the top veneer of
leadership, Sub-committee policies were implemented
by local (provincial and county) Party Committees in
infected areas, primarily in the Yangtze River Basin.
Sub-committee organizations were responsible for
mobilizing the masses and eradicating parasitic
diseases. In this organizational context, there
were virtually no regularized channels for consulting with medical and scientific organizations, as
demonstrated in Chapters 4 and 5.

Several characteristics were crucial to the
performance of the Sub-committee. First, because
its functional responsibilities were narrow (in the
sense of not being responsible for areas like medical education, research, and hospital administration), the Sub-committee could focus on parasitic
diseases. A broad range of competing interests and
perspectives which would have retarded action were
not built into its very structure. Its political
composition and its single area of responsibility
made it possible for the organization to act rapidly.

The Sub-committee's greatest virtue was also
its greatest liability. Because it could mobilize
tens of thousands of individuals rapidly, all policy
alternatives were not considered. When a program
went awry, it reached massive proportions. For
example, highly toxic drugs were administered by
untrained personnel with the result that a substantial, but unknown, number of adverse drug reactions
occurred.[8] Similarly, because the life cycle of
most parasites is extraordinarily difficult to
break, millions of days of human labor were expended
in clearing infested areas, only to find that they
easily became reinfected.[9] Finally (and this phenomenon is reappearing once again), mass antiparasite

campaigns made manpower demands on hospitals, increased patient loads in already overburdened clinical facilities, and accentuated the already acute
shortage of drugs.[10] In brief, the Sub-committee
functioned as though it was dealing with an isolated
issue area when, in fact, action in this area had a
multitude of linkages with the rest of the society.

The communes. This political arena was under
the leadership of cadres who, like those in the Sub-
committee, had no medical expertise. Because the
1958 commune was a large territorial unit, these
cadres had few ties to the local populace and even
fewer with professional organizations. Commune
Party Committees were high enough in the leadership
structure to be removed from the immediate need to
be responsive to the peasantry, and insufficiently
linked to the governmental machinery to be responsive to professional concerns.[11] Upwardly mobile
cadres often wanted "free" medical care in the communes as a tangible sign to leaders and followers
that they were advancing toward socialism. In addition, commune health centers had the appeal of providing an inducement to peasants to participate in
the communization movement. In short, commune
health centers were established to meet local needs
by individuals with no desire, or institutional
capacity, to ask what the multiplication of rural
centers meant for the health system as a whole.

The Ministry of Public Health. While antiparasite work and many rural health tasks were removed
from the Wei-sheng-pu, other areas of policy remained under its jurisdiction (e.g., higher-level
medical education, research, and hospital administration). Not only did the Ministry have specific
areas of responsibility, it was a distinctive policy-
making arena. Medical doctors were heavily represented at the organization's pinnacles. Below the
Ministry, medical schools which were directly subordinate to the Wei-sheng-pu allocated important
administrative roles to physicians, though this had
been somewhat reduced after the antirightist campaign of 1957-1958.

Within the Ministry's structure, each bureau
had its own functional area of responsibility.
Because of the interdependence of the medical field,
any policy change had to be cleared by the various
bureaucratic constituencies involved. As a result,
different interests, or concepts of the public good,
were embedded in the policy mechanism. For instance,
while the Medical Education Bureau (I-hsüeh Chiao-yü-
szu) and the Ministry of Higher Education have

255

generally pushed for the training of teachers for
medical schools, the Chinese Academy of Medical
Sciences, the Ministry's Scientific Committee of
Medical Sciences (I-hsüeh K'o-hsüeh Wei-yüan-hui),
and the Chinese Academy of Sciences have pushed for
greater emphasis upon the production of research
personnel.[12] The Treatment and Prevention Bureau
(I-liao Yü-fang-szu), in contrast to the Ministry's
research and education arms, has desired a greater
emphasis placed on the generation of public health
personnel.[13] These policy conflicts all tended to
slow the pace of change. When significant policy
departures were undertaken, they were carried out in
such a way as to minimize professional hostility and
conflict.

Implications of the divided policy-making mechanism, 1955-1960. Every policy-making system has
important advantages and disadvantages. The great
advantage of a system with several arenas was that
it enabled the total range of health programs to be
responsive to a broader range of inputs than would
have otherwise been the case. For instance, prior
to 1955, the curative health needs of China's peasant millions had not been the target of systematic
attention. With the creation of the Sub-committee
and the communes, a concerted effort was made to
meet those needs. While policy in the rural areas
was responsive to previous inequalities, the Wei-
sheng-pu was relatively more responsive to urban
needs, professional desires, and system constraints,
all of which dictated a more gradual expansion of
the manpower and organizational base. If one is
speaking in terms of the "responsive capability" of
the health system, as Almond does,[14] one would say
that it responded to the needs and desires of many
segments of the Chinese polity.

On the other hand, the divided system had important drawbacks, the most important of which was
an inability to achieve coordination. Policy emerging from one health arena had little or no logical
relationship to that emerging from another. For
instance, while the objective need for health manpower was rising rapidly (in response to the creation of commune health centers), curriculum length
in several prestigious medical schools was increased.[15] While expansion of enrollments in intermediate-level medical schools was substantial, such
increases could not have had an impact for several
years and the needs were immediate. Similarly,
expansion of drug production was not coordinated
with pharmaceutical demand. When the drug industry

256

did hastily expand production, it had to do so at the expense of quality. Finally, more referrals from rural areas vastly increased the burdens on unprepared urban hospitals.[16]

In short, the divided policy-making mechanism maximized inputs into the policy formulation process and minimized the capacity to coordinate. It was a system which evolved out of the desire to meet rural needs. A society that suffered from a pervasive limitation of resources could not long afford the costs of a system with so little capacity to coordinate.

Once the economic problems of the early 1960s descended, leaders in the communes and the Sub-committee were unable to mobilize the masses, were unable to extract the resources necessary to run commune health centers and mass campaigns, and the urban sector was reacting negatively to the perceived deterioration of municipal facilities. All these forces led to the closure of many commune health programs and the deactivation of the Sub-committee. Just as each institution had been differentially responsive to various social interests, so each arena was differentially vulnerable to severe agricultural setbacks and declines in peasant morale. In the 1961-1965 period, the system reverted to the bureaucratic configuration.

CENTRALLY-COORDINATED POLICY-MAKING, 1967-1969

The rhetoric of the Cultural Revolution projected the image of a movement designed to remove policy control from an elite and disperse those responsibilities throughout the Chinese polity. "Three-in-one revolutionary committees" were presumably one organizational vehicle by which such diffusion of authority occurred. Irrespective of the intent of the new organizations, however, important trends toward policy centralization occurred. Major directives on education, financing, and distribution of services were issued from the political system's commanding heights with little apparent consultation. Local units then had latitude in responding to these directives. There was no crucial middle-level bureaucracy that could solicit varied inputs and then give authoritative guidance to local levels during the implementation process.[17] There was centralization in policy formulation and decentralization in policy implementation; a risky combination. It led to slow implementation, lack of clarity at local levels, elite instability, and attention being given to relatively few medical issues.

The Ministry of Public Health had no visible impact upon authoritative policy in such areas as medical education, medical financing, and health delivery. During the 1967-1969 period, the few political leaders surrounding Chairman Mao Tse-tung[18] articulated the crucial health policy guidelines. The policy-making system approached Lindblom's "hierarchical" or "centrally-coordinated" model.[19] This type of policy process has certain advantages and represented both a response to the situation in 1967 and the lessons of the Great Leap Forward. It was also a system fraught with defects.

In the 1967-1969 period, not a single major health directive originated with the Wei-sheng-pu. All directives were, instead, given the imprimatur of Chairman Mao, the Central Committee, the Cultural Revolution Group, or the Standing Committee of the State Council under Chou En-lai.[20] Mao was so integral to all policy processes during this period that at least ninety-nine "latest instructions" were issued over his name. All of these had the weight of official policy.[21] Although the Chairman's most important declaration on health had actually been delivered in June 1965, it formed the touchstone for Cultural Revolution directives on medical education, the distribution of health services, and medical research.

The chief advantage of the centrally-coordinated system was its capacity to increase the level of coordination. During the Great Leap Forward, policy coordination had proven difficult to achieve due to the fragmentation of responsibilities. Excessive division of authority had precipitated unintegrated policies which, in turn, produced policy failure. In contrast, in the 1967-1969 period, areas in which policy coordination was essential (health financing, medical education, and the structure of the delivery system) were able to achieve a measure of synchronization.

The centrally-coordinated system maximized the chances that the assumptions undergirding educational policy were the same ones used in formulating directives on health delivery, and that both would be supported by appropriate financial regulations. Within the space of a few months (1968), guidelines on medical education, rural health care, and rural financing were issued. Because the directives on rural health care called for the universalization of commune and production brigade medical programs,

the elite simultaneously reduced all medical education to no longer than three years, and promulgated
directives on rural financing. Had authority been
fragmented among several political arenas, the pressures generating guidelines in each policy area
would have been different and the guidelines, themselves, would have reflected those divergences.
This did not occur. In short, the elite appears to
have learned from the Leap that medical education,
finances, and the structure of the delivery system
were all highly interdependent.

The centrally-coordinated apparatus had important defects. These blemishes have necessitated
changes in the structure of the post-Cultural Revolution policy-making system. The major problem with
this system was that it limited the inputs which
members of the elite could take into account.
Because the elite was composed of individuals bur-
dened with more responsibilities than either time
or capacities to handle, they could only consider a
small percentage of the data which were relevant to
any given decision. Two things followed: First,
the range of policy was limited to a few functional
areas (e.g., medical education, financing, and
health delivery). Only in that way could policy-
makers consider at least the most relevant data
bearing on decisions. Secondly, as the elite's
policy responsibilities proliferated, directives
issued in one area tended to produce unintended
consequences in others.

In what ways were these difficulties evident?
The most notable attribute of this period was that
very few areas of medical policy actually received
attention. While directives were issued on medical
education, financing, and rural health care, there
were no guidelines on medical research, mass campaigns, professional life, or the role of professional associations. In fact, policy in these areas
only began to emerge in 1973,[22] as part of a more
generalized movement away from the Cultural Revolution. Of course, the areas in which directives were
first issued were the most urgent, but policy uncertainty in research, for instance, spilled over into
medical education where professors were unsure of
their role.

Unintended consequences have resulted from
policies which, had they been made in a broader
forum, might have been modified. For instance,
barefoot doctors have often become vehicles for
referring more patients to urban hospitals.[23] Instead of lightening the burdens on these facilities

(as they were supposed to do) they have frequently
increased them by finding more disease than many
localities are able to treat. Had the elite tapped
the experience of prior vice-ministers of public
health, as it related to their knowledge of the
first barefoot doctors program (1958), they could
have anticipated the problems which, once again,
are evident.

Because the major decision-makers were few, the
values of this small group were crucial. This meant
that even small changes in elite composition could
produce drastic alterations in policy. This had two
consequences: First, subordinate agencies had
little expectation that policy would remain stable.
This encouraged local administrators to be wary in
implementing programs and to move cautiously in the
absence of very explicit instructions. One example
of this phenomenon related to agricultural mechanization.

> In the absence of directives from the higher
> level and without experience, we are afraid
> that in the event of trouble the responsibility
> would be too heavy for anybody. It would be
> better to wait for directives from the higher
> level.[24]

In short, when policies were not fully spelled out,
implementation was slower than would have otherwise
been the case. This was particularly apparent in
medical education; 1968 directives were not opera-
tionalized until 1971. While there were many reasons for this glacial rate of movement, one factor
was that local administrators and teachers feared
to implement policies which could subsequently be
criticized if a shift occurred at the unstable top.[25]
In short, bureaucracy provides one thing lower-level
participants badly need--predictability.

An additional result of having a centrally-
coordinated policy-making apparatus was that because
so few persons had so much impact on programs, a
premium was placed on being one of those individuals.
Because power was concentrated, it made a great deal
of difference who held the reins. This aggravated
leadership instability, a condition still further
exacerbated by the need to define procedures for
determining the succession to Chairman Mao. The
results of these tensions surfaced in 1970-1971 with
the purge of Ch'en Po-ta and the attempt of Lin Piao
to seize power.[26] No sooner had Lin been purged
than prolonged conflict broke out between the elite

beneficiaries of the Cultural Revolution and its elite victims.[27] At issue was how much of the Cultural Revolution legacy should be preserved and how many of the movement's victims should remain purged? This conflict came to a head in 1976 with the January death of Premier Chou En-lai and the September passing of Mao. The military ultimately sided with those in favor of more conventional educational and developmental policies, most notably Hua Kuo-feng. This, in turn, resulted in the somewhat indelicate vilification of Mao's widow and her three "radical" allies, collectively dubbed the "gang of four."

In sum, the movement of policy-making power to the top of the political system, and the concurrent decentralization of policy implementation authority, had three consequences: it made local initiative risky, increased elite instability, and limited the scope of policy.

The preceding discussion contains several propositions about the sources of recent changes in the centrally-coordinated system. First of all, because the central elite had limited information processing capabilities, it was unable to make policy in as many areas as modern health systems require. This is part of the reason why policy vis à vis medical research and professional life only began to appear in 1972-1973. Secondly, strong countervailing pressures were (and are) built in for delegation of authority away from the Center. Policy-making responsibilities are acquired in the course of program implementation. Because a small elite is unable to make all policy decisions for more than a short period, there is a tendency toward delegation of authority. To say, however, that policy responsibilities tend to become more widely dispersed is not to say that such powers necessarily devolve to "the people," whoever they may be defined as being. The most likely repository for such authority, in the Chinese case, is the bureaucracy.[28]

THE RECURRING BUREAUCRATIC POLICY-MAKING SYSTEM

Had this chapter proceeded chronologically, it would have first analyzed this policy-making system. From the very opening days of the People's Republic, the Ministry of Public Health assumed substantial responsibilities. By necessity, if not design, the Wei-sheng-pu was run by medical doctors, trained abroad and dedicated to science and quality medicine, as well as mass-oriented medical care. In periods

261

after heroic efforts had been made to reduce the impact and/or autonomy of the Wei-sheng-pu, the Ministry invariably reemerged as the single most important source of medical policy. The "equilibrium" nature of the bureaucratic system derives from the basic instabilities of the divided and centrally-coordinated policy-making systems. As we have seen, however, the bureaucratic system is subject to destabilizations of its own.

The Ministry of Public Health has been the primary site of medical policy-making for approximately nineteen of the last twenty-eight years, with elite decision-makers in the Party and government hierarchies frequently assuming the role of referee. As decisions have become progressively more complex, and the Party and state elite more functionally specialized and fragmented itself,[29] lines of cleavage at the Center have increasingly paralleled the fissures in the bureaucracy and society at large.

Because the Ministry has so frequently been the primary site of health policy-making, the political and organizational matrix in which it has been embedded, its internal structure, and its leadership have been the most important variables in explaining policy.

The Ministry of Public Health is a bureaucratic organization consisting of at least a dozen bureaus (in Peking) and similar structures in each provincial-level unit and county. The more specialized the bureau, the more dominant professionals have been, at least during those periods for which we have detailed information.[30] Bureaucratic conflict has been the result of division of responsibility within such a complex organization. When the analyst takes the Ministry's relationship to subordinate health departments in the provinces, cities, and counties into consideration, the picture of conflict comes into still starker relief. The Ministry has repeatedly tried to get local hospitals and clinics to provide more services while, at the same time, attempting to minimize its own financial liabilities.

Bureaucratic tensions have not only been apparent among Ministry bureaus and between levels in the health system, they have also been evident between the central Party elite and the Ministry leadership. The Center has sporadically directed the Wei-sheng-pu to provide additional services to the populace, but has been reluctant to increase budgetary allocations commensurately. This was conspicuously the case when Minister Ch'ien Hsin-chung asked Teng Hsiao-p'ing for increased funding prior to the

Cultural Revolution.[31] In short, the Wei-sheng-pu
is an organization in which many interests converge.
Because of the tugging and hauling, policy consensus
is difficult to achieve and, once achieved, resistant to alteration. Policy emerging from this context has tended to be evolutionary, not revolutionary.

Every policy-making system has its own strengths
and weaknesses. The bureaucratic system's capacity
to achieve program coordination may not be as great
as the centrally-coordinated system's,[32] but it is
certainly superior to the divided system's capabilities in this regard. This is so because many issue
areas related to health care are under some degree
of Ministry influence. In the cases where this has
not been true, and issues have cut across ministries,
conflict has occurred and progress has been stalled.
For instance, the Wei-sheng-pu has periodically had
difficulty persuading other agencies to lower pharmaceutical prices. Similarly, industrial health
work, because of the need for substantial outside
cooperation, has not been notably successful.[33]
Finally, environmental protection has been an area
where the Ministry has found it difficult to gain
the full cooperation of outside organizations. In
sum, the bureaucratic system does not do away with
overlapping jurisdictions, but it does keep them
within tolerable limits. The coordination capacity
that has been achieved has been gained without excessive reliance upon a small elite.

In the discussion of the divided system, we
observed that its greatest attribute was its capacity to respond to a broad range of societal needs
and demands. The major difficulty was that not all
societal needs could be met simultaneously and, yet,
there was no forum in which integrative decisions
were made and priorities established. By comparison, the bureaucratic system is less likely to
generate policies responsive to widely divergent
inputs. At the same time, it is able to cope with
a broader range of inputs than the centrally-coordinated system.

What leads one to believe that the above is
true? First, the health bureaucracy can gather and
process more conflicting data than a small elite
because: (1) The Wei-sheng-pu is not concerned with
the range of issues which confront the national
elite. (2) The Ministry has more personnel to analyze data. (3) The Ministry is a complex organization in which various social interests have been
institutionalized.

While the bureaucratic system can cope with a
broader range of inputs than the centrally-coordinated type, some interests and perspectives have been
expressed "more equally" than others. The health
bureaucracy does not afford equal access to all,[34]
and the mere fact of access does not assure that all
perspectives are equally effective. The Wei-sheng-
pu has given physicians a strong institutional position at the bureau and vice-ministerial levels,
while rural perspectives have been slighted. The
reasons for this seem to stem from the fact that
while medical professionals are a relatively coherent entity in terms of values, interests, and needs,
peasants are not. Relatively well-to-do peasants
often prefer to go to urban facilities while poorer
and more remote inhabitants frequently favor lower
cost, cooperative, and convenient health services.[35]
Similarly, peasants in one locale may be faced with
diseases which are all but irrelevant to inhabitants
of another area. In short, peasant interests are
not as homogeneous as those of physicians.

Leaders of large urban areas (e.g., P'eng Chen)
have also been in a relatively strong position to
influence health policy[36] by inhibiting the Center
from exerting pressure on the Wei-sheng-pu to transfer medical resources to distant rural areas.[37]
Their strength derives from several sources, the
most important of which is the fact that big medical
facilities are already in the cities. As well,
insured cadres and workers are concentrated in
urban centers. In the political tugging and hauling,
prevailing interests, efficiency, and strategic
location predispose the Ministry to be relatively
more responsive to urban problems.

For all these reasons, the conclusion that the
bureaucratic system handles a broader range of inputs than the centrally-coordinated system is not to
be confused with saying that a bureaucratic structure is the most equitable form of organization
imaginable. In fact, it was these inequities which
Chairman Mao tried to overcome twice: once by
lifting certain issue areas from the bureaucracy
and once by temporarily emasculating the Ministry.

POLITICAL CHANGE IN CHINA: TOWARD A FRAMEWORK

Having identified changes in the structure of
the Chinese health policy-making apparatus, we must
ask, what have been the forces generating these
alterations? The basic explanation derives from

the proposition that every policy-making system alienates certain groups or individuals and meets the minimal demands of others. In analyzing system change, one has to assess the relative strengths of disgruntled sectors of the society and leadership and the role that policy outputs play in generating financial and administrative pressures for change. Because we have proposed that the bureaucratic system has been an "equilibrium" form, we ought to describe briefly the forces which periodically have rendered it unstable.

The major reasons for departure from the "equilibrium" state have been due to what might be called the effects of Merton and Mao. As Robert Merton noted, high-level administrators in bureaucratic organizations demand predictable and regularized behavior from lower participants. This predictability tends to be interpreted as rigidity by clients.

> The reduction in personalized relationships, the increased internalization of rules, and the decreased search for alternatives combine to make the behavior of members of the organization highly predictable, i.e., they result in an increase in the rigidity of behavior . . . [this] facilitates the development of an esprit de corps. . . . Such a sense of commonness of purpose, interests, and character increases the propensity of an organization member to defend each other against outside pressures. . . . [This creates] client disaffection.[38]

The very nature of the health bureaucracy generates hostilities among its clients.

Added to this basic level of social hostility is the fact that health resources have been extraordinarily scarce. The need to allocate has meant in practice that certain sectors of the society will receive greater benefits than others. As we have repeatedly noted, not more than 25 percent of the urban population has access to free health services, and the quality of attention has, to some extent, been dependent upon one's status. Mao openly acknowledged these inequities and these cleavages provided the basis for his successive political strategies in 1958 and 1966.

The simple existence of hostility, however, is insufficient alone to account for system change. First of all, allocation is imperative and sectors of the society which would be hurt by any reallocation of services have resisted (and can be expected

to continue to resist) changes which would be to
their detriment. Urban leaders have tended to
resist redistributive proposals.[39] Most importantly,
diffuse social discontent will not produce change
unless it is legitimized and channeled. During his
lifetime, Mao played a pivotal role in this regard.[40] The kind of interventionist role which the
Chairman played in the Great Leap, however, was
quite different from the one he assumed during the
Cultural Revolution.

In 1955, Mao adopted an essentially preemptive
strategy in an attempt to meet the needs of neglected
sectors of the population, most notably the peasantry. Several events convinced the Chairman that
the problems were worthy of attention. First, the
Hungarian revolt (and the difficulties in Poland)
demonstrated what the results of unattended discontent could be. Secondly, the Soviet-style developmental program was not generating sufficiently rapid
growth or fostering patterns of distribution which
would nurture the belief that the inequalities would
be corrected as a matter of course. Initially, Mao
was willing to make concessions to the intellectuals
in order to gain their support and cooperation in
correcting some of the social and economic problems
which he felt could rip Chinese society asunder.[41]
With the "inappropriate" response of the intellectuals (mid-1957), the Chairman was forced to adopt
a new strategy; rely upon the "masses" by expanding
the scope of organizations in which they could play
a decisive role (e.g., the Nine Man Sub-committee).
The Great Leap, then, was not so much an attack upon
established institutions as it was an assertion that
new organizations could meet previously unmet needs.

Mao's role in the Cultural Revolution was far
different. Then he consciously mobilized the disenchanted sectors of the society to attack the entire bureaucracy and Party. The Chairman was now
operating well outside the "rules of the game."
Disaffected students, persons who resented the
favored treatment accorded cadres, workers excluded
from benefits, and some suburban peasants were all
mobilized. Concurrent with this emasculation of the
Ministry, Mao, and a small group around him, became
the major source of authoritative policy. The crucial difference between the Great Leap and the Cultural Revolution was that the disaffection mobilized
in the Leap was used to proliferate the number of
institutions; in the Cultural Revolution, disaffec-
tions were mobilized to temporarily eliminate the
bureaucratic middle level.

A LAST WORD

   This study has outlined a process of political
development spanning twenty-eight years. The major
factors shaping that process throughout this period
have been popular perceptions of inequalities, Mao's
willingness (and capacity) to play a mobilizational
role, and the administrative problems which emerged
when a new pattern of policy-making arenas was
created. While Mao's death eliminates one of these
major variables, policy will still reflect the enduring importance of the divisive need to allocate
and the unanticipated consequences which inevitably
flow from policy actions. A primary uncertainty for
the future is whether or not individual leaders, or
groups of them, will have the capability or desire
to mobilize disgruntled sectors of the society on
their behalf.   There is reason to think that this
mobilizational feature may be less conspicuous with
the passing of Mao, the one political figure who
possessed both the capacity and legitimacy to do this.
   We conclude that there has been a tendency
toward an optimizing health policy-making system.
Optimizing does not mean the "best," but merely a
process which can produce policy coordination and
simultaneously take a decent range of inputs into
account. The real question for the future is whether
or not an increasingly broad range of interests will
become institutionalized in the bureaucracy, especially rural perspectives. If this occurs, the
primary achievement of the Chinese experiment may
well be seen as being the construction of a health
bureaucracy in which a relatively broad range of
interests are embedded.

NOTES

1.   "P'i-p'ing Ho Ch'eng T'ung-chih Tsai Tui-tai
Chung-i Te Cheng-t'se-shang Te Ts'o-wu" [Criticize
Comrade Ho Ch'eng's mistakes with respect to the
treatment of traditional Chinese medicine], Jen-min
Jih-pao [People's daily], November 20, 1955.

2.   "National Antischistosomiasis Meeting Convened
in Shanghai," Kuang-ming Jih-pao [Bright daily],
April 7, 1956.

3.   "All China Conference on Parasitic Diseases,"
Chinese Medical Journal 77 (1958):519.

4. Central-coordination is discussed in Charles E. Lindblom, _The Intelligence of Democracy_ (New York: Free Press, 1965).

5. David M. Lampton, "Trends in Health Policy," _Current Scene_ 12, no. 6 (June 1974):1-9. In retrospect, the Second Plenum of the Ninth Central Committee (August-September 1970) may be seen as an important turning point. The Tenth National Congress of the Chinese Communist Party (August 1973) certainly was a landmark, as well.

6. Mao Tse-tung, "Preface to Socialist Upsurge in China's Countryside," _Hsin Jen Wei_ [New people's health] (Peking: People's Health Press, 1967), in _Survey of China Mainland Magazines-Supplement_ (hereafter _SCMM-S_), no. 22, pp. 9-10.

7. By 1958, one's degree of medical expertise was inversely correlated with one's influence upon Subcommittee decisions. In May 1958 (_People's Daily_, May 16, 1958), Wei Wen-po attacked medical experts for being conservative and obstructionist when plans for the rapid elimination of schistosomiasis were being formulated.

8. David M. Lampton, _Interview Files 21 C and 21 E_. Confirmation of this is suggested by _Chung-hua I-hsüeh Tsa-chih_ [Chinese medical journal], no. 1 (1974), pp. 1-2. In this article on cardiac pacemakers, the author notes that Adams-Stokes syndrome (atrioventricular block) had resulted from high dosages of antimony. Antimony was administered in high dosages in the treatment of schistosomiasis during the Great Leap Forward. During my October 1976 visit to a Shanghai hospital, a doctor confirmed that high dosages of antimony had been associated with cardiac problems.

9. _Jen-min Jih-pao_ [People's daily], January 24, 1964, noted, ". . . schistosomiasis affects wide areas, and the factors for its outbreak are very complicated. Those who have been cured of this disease may be affected by it again. It is impossible to wipe out all snails within a short time. . . ." See _Survey of the China Mainland Press_ hereafter _SCMP_), no. 3160, p. 5.

10. Hangchow, Chekiang Provincial Service in Mandarin, February 27, 1974, in _Foreign Broadcast Information Service, Daily Report: People's Republic of China_ (hereafter _FBIS_), no. 53 (1974), p. C 3.

11. Franz Schurmann, Ideology and Organization in Communist China (Berkeley: University of California Press, 1968), pp. 193-194.

12. Yang Hsiu-feng, "Higher Education in China," New China News Agency (hereafter NCNA), June 20, 1956, in Current Background (hereafter CB), no. 400, p. 16.

13. Chien-k'ang Pao [Health bulletin], May 7, 1957.

14. Gabriel Almond and Bingham Powell, Comparative Politics: A Developmental Approach (Boston: Little, Brown and Company, 1966), pp. 201-203.

15. "Thoroughly Criticize and Repudiate the Eight-Year Medical Education Program Pushed by China's Khrushchev," China's Medicine 3 (1968):164-169.

16. David M. Lampton, Interview File 21 E; see also, Ezra Vogel, Interviews Nos. 8 and 19; see also, Hangchow, Chekiang Provincial Service in Mandarin, February 27, 1974, in FBIS, no. 53 (1974), pp. C 2-C 3, for similar problems in the 1970s.

17. Donald S. Van Meter and Carl E. Van Horn, "The Policy Implementation Process: Intergovernmental Relations and Social Policies" (Delivered at the 1974 Annual Meeting of the American Political Science Association, Chicago, Illinois, August 29-September 2, 1974).

18. While the precise composition of this group cannot be fully assessed in the absence of full knowledge about the policy process at this level, Mao, Chou En-lai, Lin Piao, Ch'en Po-ta, K'ang Sheng, and Chiang Ch'ing all played crucial roles.

19. Lindblom, Part 5.

20. In order to get a feeling for the centralization of authority characteristic of this period see, CCP Documents of the Great Proletarian Cultural Revolution 1966-1967 (Hong Kong: Union Research Institute, 1968), pp. 1-27.

21. E. L. Wheelwright and Bruce McFarlane, The Chinese Road to Socialism (New York: Monthly Review Press, 1970), pp. 227-240.

22. Only by 1973 had Chung-hua I-hsüeh Tsa-chih [Chinese medical journal] resumed publication and

had the Chinese Medical Association regained some of its pre-Cultural Revolution visibility.

23. Hangchow, Chekiang Provincial Service in Mandarin, February 27, 1974, in FBIS, no. 53 (1974), pp. C 2-C 3; see also, South China Morning Post, February 1, 1973, p. 13.

24. "March with Big Strides on the Revolutionary Road--How Chengting Hsien Station's Farm Machines and Tools Were Sent Down," in Selections From China Mainland Magazines (hereafter SCMM), no. 643, p. 8. This was cited by Benedict Stavis, "Mechanical Power to the People: Decentralization of Management of Agricultural Machinery in China." (Presented at the American Society of Public Administration's 1974 National Conference, Syracuse, New York, May 5-8, 1974), p. 59. While Stavis does not fully share my views on the general issue of concentration of power during the Cultural Revolution, it does appear that the phenomena he noted are compatible with my interpretation.

25. A 1974 broadcast demonstrates how policy and personnel instabilities affect the willingness of lower participants to assume responsibilities. (See Ch'engchow, Honan Provincial Service in Mandarin, FBIS, no. 51 (1974), p. D 1.) "However, . . . having been criticized, a situation has evolved in which some teachers do not concern themselves with things emerging from among the students that are incompatible with Mao Tse-tung Thought. . . . They just want to push responsibility onto student cadres so that they themselves will not be held responsible."

26. "Pre-Anniversary Purge of 'May 16' Elements," China News Summary (hereafter CNS), no. 374, pp. A 1-A 4; see also, "Purged and Dropped Members of CCP Ninth Central Committee," CNS, no. 484, Part 3; see also, "Ch'en Po-ta Publicly Denounced," CNS, no. 391, pp. A 1-A 2; see also, "Lin Piao's Crimes," CNS, no. 404, pp. 1-13.

27. This was a fascinating period which witnessed the 1973 resurrection of Teng Hsiao-p'ing, the Cultural Revolution's second most famous victim. Along with Teng's return, increasing numbers of pre-Cultural Revolution ministers returned to important posts. These trends, in turn, fueled the complex "Anti-Confucian Campaign" of 1973-1974. See, Merle Goldman, "China's Anti-Confucian Campaign, 1973-1974," China Quarterly, no. 63 (1975), pp. 435-462.

28. Milovan Djilas, The New Class (New York: Praeger, 1957). Djilas argues that this is approximately what happened in the Soviet Union.

29. A. Doak Barnett, Cadres, Bureaucracy, and Political Power in Communist China (New York: Columbia University Press, 1967), pp. 3-10.

30. Ezra Vogel, Interview No. 42.

31. "Mayflies Lightly Plot to Topple Giant Tree," Ch'üan-wu-ti [Invincible] (June 26, 1967), in SCMP-S, no. 209, p. 21.

32. Charles Lindblom would argue that a "partisan mutual bargaining" system has a greater capacity for coordination.

33. David M. Lampton, Wingspread Report: Health Care in the People's Republic Of China (Racine, Wisconsin: The Johnson Foundation, 1973), p. 16.

34. David Truman, The Governmental Process (New York: Alfred A. Knopf, 1971). Truman devotes considerable space to showing how some interests are more strategically located for influencing one segment of the governmental machinery than another.

35. "Rural Cooperative Medical Service," CB, no. 872, pp. 1-42.

36. David M. Lampton, Interview File 21 E.

37. "Mayflies Lightly Plot to Topple Giant Tree," p. 22.

38. James G. March and Herbert A. Simon, Organizations (New York: Wiley & Sons, Incorporated, 1966), p. 39. March and Simon elaborate on Merton's ideas at length.

39. As P'eng Chen said, "Only after the cities have been put in order . . . can we proceed to work the rural villages." Ch'üan-wu-ti [Invincible] (June 26, 1967), in SCMP-S, no. 209, p. 22.

40. Michel Oksenberg, "Policy-Making Under Mao Tsetung, 1949-1968," Comparative Politics 3, no. 3 (1971):323-359.

41. Roderick MacFarquhar, <u>The Origins of the Cul-</u>
<u>tural Revolution: Contradictions Among the People,</u>
<u>1956-1957</u> (New York: Columbia University Press,
1974). MacFarquhar very clearly shows that Mao was
the major force pushing for "open door rectification"
throughout late 1956 and early 1957. The Chairman
was relatively optimistic about the utility of
intellectuals in rectifying Party and social defects.

APPENDIXES

Appendix A
Table of Ministry Organization

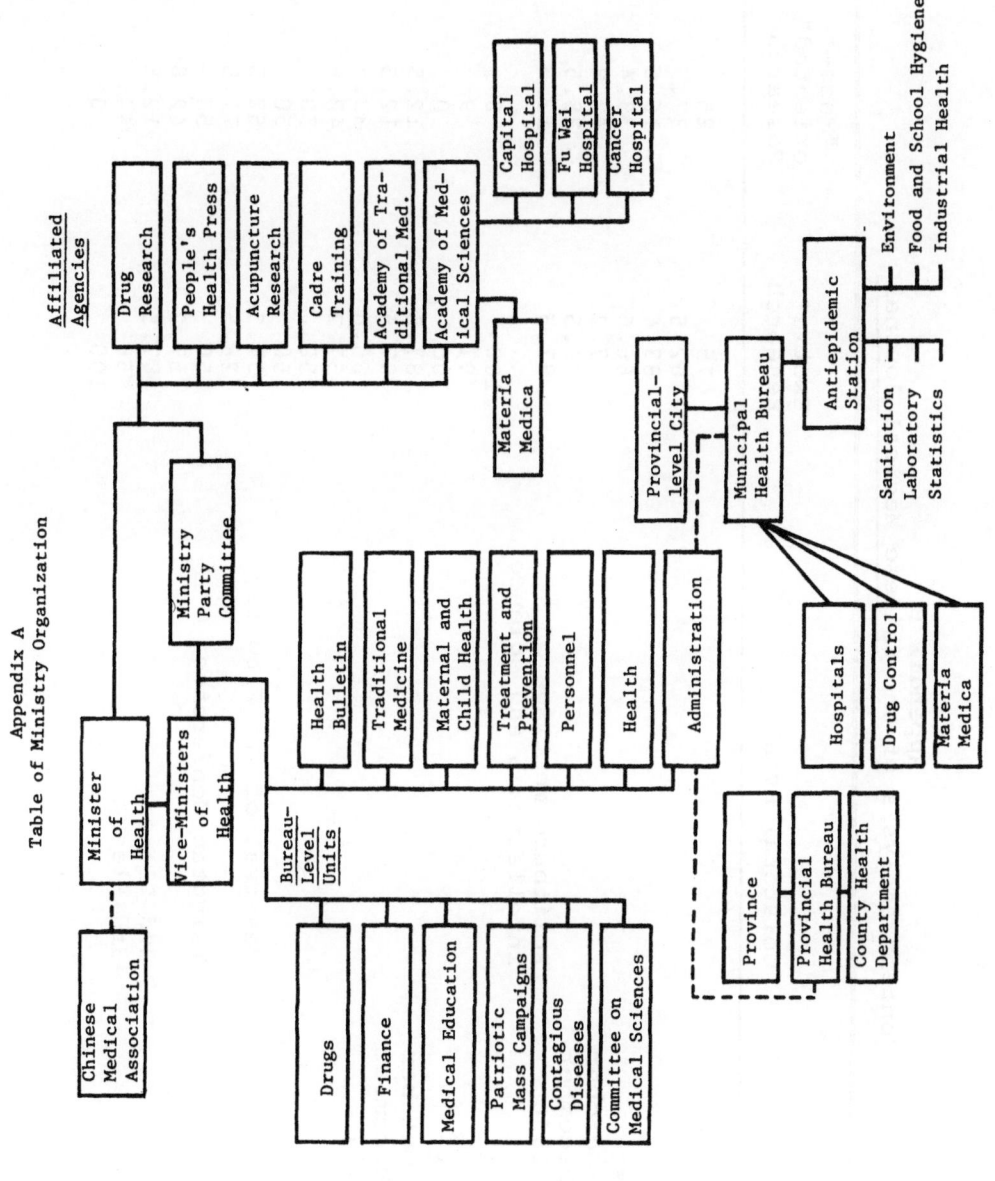

275

Appendix B

Content Analysis of the Chinese Medical Journal

Date	Colateral Event	Exotic* Research	"Mass-*oriented" Research
Jan.-Feb. 1955		75	25
March-April		62.5	37.5
May-June		83.4	16.6
July-August		66.6	33.4
September-October		57.2	42.8
November-December		71.5	28.5
Jan.-Feb. 1956		87.5	12.5
March-April	Politburo meetings on intellectuals and science	100	0
May-June		91	9
July-August		100	0
September-October		87.5	12.5
November-December		87.5	12.5
January 1957		66.6	33.4
February		57.2	42.8
March		50	50
April		50	50
May	Reversal of 100 Flowers	37.5	62.5
June		28.5	71.5
July	Tsingtao Conference	50	50
August		57.2	42.8
September	3rd Plenum	87.5	12.5
October	3rd Plenum	56	44
November		100	0

Appendix B Continued.

Date	Colateral Event	Exotic* Research	"Mass-*oriented" Research
December		66.6	33.4
January 1958	Hangchow and Nanning Meetings	14.4	85.6
February		71.5	28.5
March	Ch'engtu Meeting	62.5	37.5
April		50	50
May	2nd Session, 8th Central	75	25
June	Committee and 4th and 5th Plenums	91	9
July		55	45
August	Peitaiho Conference, communes	46	54
September		66.6	33.4
October		72.8	27.3
November	1st Chengchow Meeting, Wuchang Meeting and 6th Plenum	70	30
December	Mao steps down	20	80
January 1959	Politburo Conference	30	70
February	2nd Chengchow Conference	42.8	57.2
March	2nd Chengchow Conference	75	25
April	7th Plenum	75	25
May		63.7	36.3
June		50	50
July		50	50
August	8th Plenum	79	21

Appendix B Continued.

Date	Colateral Event	Exotic* Research	"Mass-* oriented" Research
September-October		87.5	12.5
November		71.5	28.5
December		60	40
January 1960		11	89
February		61	39
March		63	37
April		54	46
May		50	50
June		60	40

Remainder of year 1960 and all of 1961 were not available.

*The operational definition of "exotic" research is slippery in many cases, but "exotic" articles deal with problems that are: (a) relatively rare, (b) require elaborate and costly treatment which only a few specialists can accomplish, and (c) are of greater concern to the international medical community than the immediate clinical needs of China. The usual "exotic" research article begins by stating, "While we have only seen four cases of this problem in the last ten years, it is intrinsically interesting because. . ." Since the categories are loose, however, the margin of "error" in the content analysis is substantial. This table appeared in David M. Lampton, "Health Policy During the Great Leap Forward," China Quarterly, no. 60 (1974), pp. 672-673.

Appendix C
RED GUARD ORGANIZATIONS

Name	First Known Appearance
1. Ministry of Health Revolutionary Committee.	February 28, 1967
2. Preparatory Committee of the Ministry of Health Red Rebel Committee.	March 1967
3. Peking Academy of Sciences Long March Red Guard Spark Commune.	
4. Capital Hospital Revolutionary Committee.	May 1967
5. Chien-k'ang Pao Yenan Commune.	Early 1967
6. Revolutionary Liaison.	March 1967
7. The East is Red.	circa March 1967
8. The People's Servant.	circa March 1967
9. Hsin Yun Shui-nu.	circa March 1967
10. Long Spear in Hand.	circa March 1967
11. Red Rebels.	circa March 1967
12. The Spark Commune.	circa May 1967
13. The Red Representatives of China Medical College Red Flag Commune.	circa May 1967

Name	First Known Appearance
14. The Ministry of Public Health Red Corps.	circa May 1967
15. The Root Out Huang Shu-ts'e Combat Corps.	circa June 1967
16. The Red Representatives of Peking Academy of Traditional Chinese Medicine Red Flag Combat Corps.	circa June 1967
17. Revolutionary Committee of Grand Alliances of Peking Medical and Health Circles.	
18. August 18 Joint Headquarters of Peking Medical College Red Guard Congress.	
19. Peking Municipal Health Department Red Rebels.	circa August 1967 (?)

Appendix D

Number of Medical Conferences Held and Attended by Chinese*

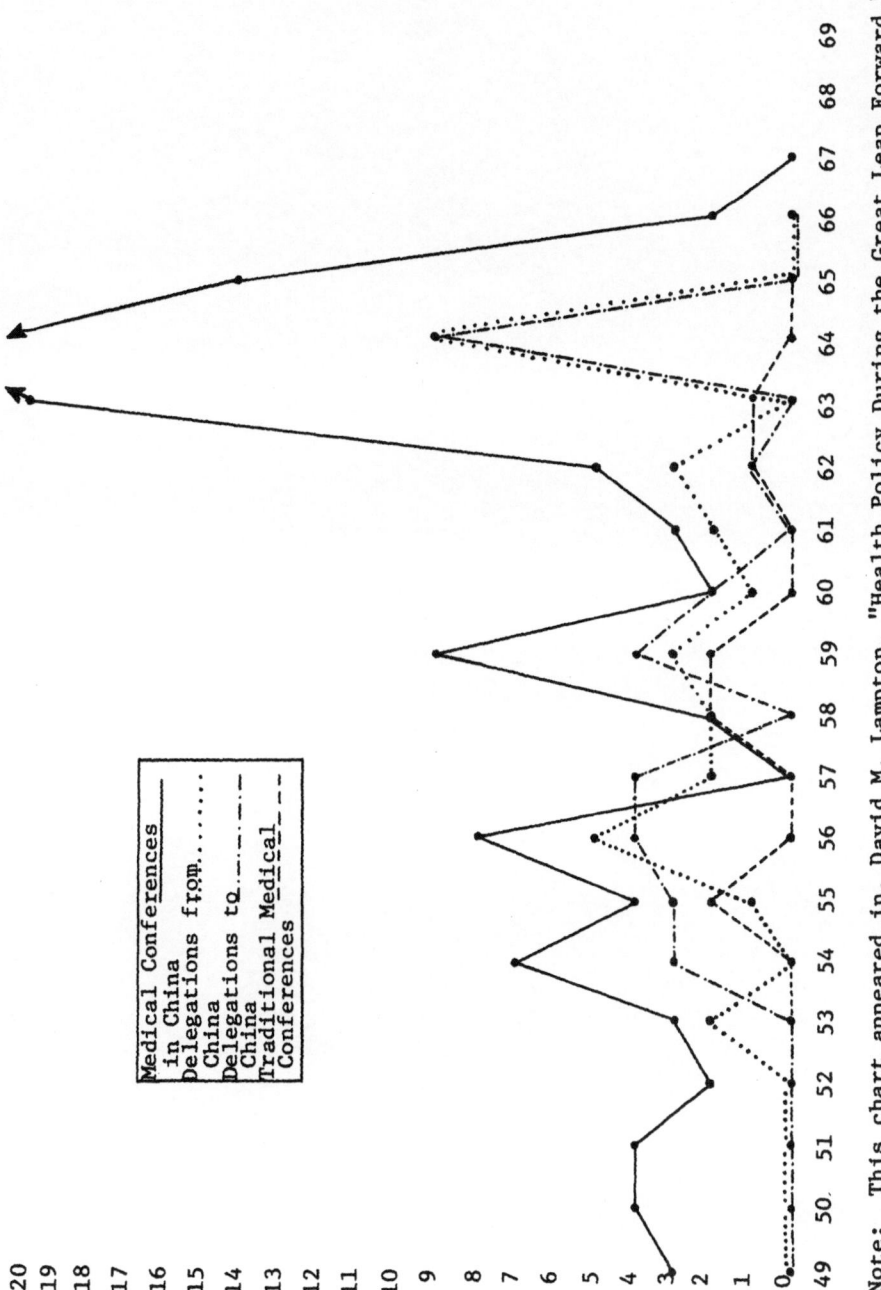

Note: This chart appeared in, David M. Lampton, "Health Policy During the Great Leap Forward," _China Quarterly_, no. 60 (1974), p. 671.

281

SELECTED BIBLIOGRAPHY

SELECTED BIBLIOGRAPHY

ARTICLES

Aird, John S. "Population Policy and Demographic Prospects in the People's Republic of China." People's Republic of China: An Economic Assessment. Washington, D.C.: Joint Economic Committee, 1972.

Alley, Rewi. "Life and Industrial Growth in Wusih." Eastern Horizon 10, no. 4 (1971):17-26.

Baum, Richard. "The Cultural Revolution in the Countryside: Anatomy of a Limited Rebellion." The Cultural Revolution in China. Edited by Thomas W. Robinson. Berkeley: University of California Press, 1971.

Berger, Roland. "Medical Training in China." Eastern Horizon 12, no. 1 (1973):28-36. Entire issue deals with medicine in China.

Bernstein, Thomas P. "Cadre and Peasant Behavior Under Conditions of Insecurity and Deprivation: The Grain Supply Crisis of the Spring of 1955." Chinese Communist Politics in Action. Edited by A. Doak Barnett. Seattle: University of Washington Press, 1969.

_____. "Leadership and Mass Mobilisation in the Soviet and Chinese Collectivisation Campaigns of 1929-30 and 1955-56: A Comparison." China Quarterly, no. 31 (1967):1-47.

Bowers, John Z. "The History of Public Health in China to 1937." Public Health in the People's Republic of China. Edited by Myron E. Wegman, Tsung-yi Lin, and Elizabeth F. Purcell. New York: The Josiah Macy, Jr. Foundation, 1973.

_____. "Medicine in Mainland China: Red and
     Rural." Current Scene 3, no. 12 (1970).

Chandra-sekhar, Sripati. "Marx, Malthus and Mao:
     China's Population Explosion." Current Scene
     5, no. 3 (1967):1-14.

Chen, William. "Medicine and Public Health." China
     Quarterly, no. 6 (1961):153-164.

_____. "Medicine and Public Health in China
     Today." Public Health Reports 76, no. 8 (1961):
     699-708.

Cheng Chu-yuan. "Health Manpower: Growth and Distri-
     bution." Public Health in the People's Repub-
     lic of China. Edited by Myron E. Wegman, Tsung-
     yi Lin, and Elizabeth F. Purcell. New York:
     The Josiah Macy, Jr. Foundation, 1973.

Cheng Tien-hsi. "Schistosomiasis in Mainland China."
     American Journal of Tropical Medicine and
     Hygiene 20, no. 1 (1971):26-53.

"China's Medical Services: Mao's Thought in Opera-
     tion." China News Summary, no. 231 (1968):7-9.

"The Conflict Between Mao Tse-tung and Liu Shao-ch'i
     Over Agricultural Mechanization in Communist
     China." Current Scene 6, no. 17 (1968).

Dimond, E. Grey. "Acupuncture Anesthesia." Journal
     of the American Medical Association 218, no. 10
     (1971):1558-1563.

_____. "Medical Education and Care in People's
     Republic of China." Journal of the American
     Medical Association 218, no. 10 (1971):1552-
     1557.

_____. "Medical School Curriculum in the
     People's Republic of China." Journal of the
     American Medical Association 236, no. 13 (1976):
     1489-1491.

Djerassi, Carl. "Fertility Limitation Through Con-
     traceptive Steroids in the People's Republic
     of China." Studies in Family Planning 5, no. 1
     (1974):13-30.

Eckstein, Alexander. "Economic Growth and Change in China: A Twenty-Year Perspective." *China Quarterly*, no. 54 (1973):211-241.

Gardner, John. "Educated Youth and Urban-Rural Inequalities, 1958-66." *The City in Communist China*. Edited by John Wilson Lewis. Stanford: Stanford University Press, 1971.

George, Alexander L. "The 'Operational Code': A Neglected Approach to the Study of Political Leaders and Decision-making." *International Studies Quarterly* 13, no. 2 (1969):190-222.

Goldman, Merle. "Party Policies Toward the Intellectuals: The Unique Blooming and Contending of 1961-2." *Party Leadership and Revolutionary Power in China*. Edited by John Wilson Lewis. London: Cambridge University Press, 1970.

_____. "China's Anti-Confucian Campaign, 1973-74." *China Quarterly*, no. 63 (1975):435-462.

Goss, Mary. "Influence and Authority Among Physicians in an Out-patient Clinic." *Complex Organizations*. Edited by Amitai Etzioni. New York: Free Press, 1961.

Harper, Paul. "The Party and the Unions in Communist China." *China Quarterly*, no. 37 (1969): 84-119.

Hough, Jerry. "The Party Apparatchiki." *Interest Groups in Soviet Politics*. Edited by H. Gordon Skilling and Franklyn Griffiths. Princeton: Princeton University Press, 1971.

I-hsüeh Shih Yü Pao-chien Tsu-chih [Medical history and health organization] 1 (1958).

"Interview with Chinese Medical Doctor." *Current Scene* 1, no. 3 (1961):1-12.

Israel, John. "The Red Guards in Historical Perspective: Continuity and Change in the Chinese Youth Movement." *China Quarterly*, no. 30 (1967):1-32.

Lampton, David M. "Economics, Politics, and the Determinants of Policy Outcomes in China: Post-Cultural Revolution Health Policy." *The*

Australian and New Zealand Journal of Sociology
12, no. 1 (1976):43-49.

_____. "Health Care in the People's Republic
of China." _Wingspread Report_ (November 1973).

_____. "Health Policy During the Great Leap
Forward." _China Quarterly_, no. 60 (1974):668-
698.

_____. "Policy Arenas and the Study of Chinese
Politics." _Studies in Comparative Communism_
7, no. 4 (1974):409-413.

_____. "Public Health and Politics in China's
Past Two Decades." _Health Services Reports_ 87,
no. 10 (1972):895-904.

_____. "Trends in Health Policy." _Current
Scene_ 12, no. 6 (1974):1-9.

Lardy, Nicholas R. "Centralization and Decentralization in China's Fiscal Management." _China
Quarterly_, no. 61 (1975):25-60.

Lewis, John Wilson. "Commerce, Education, and
Political Development in Tangshan, 1956-69."
The City in Communist China. Edited by John W.
Lewis. Stanford: Stanford University Press,
1971.

_____. "Leader, Commissar, and Bureaucrat:
The Chinese Political System in the Last Days
of the Revolution." _China in Crisis_. Edited
by Ho Ping-ti and Tsou Tang. 1, no. 2.
Chicago: University of Chicago Press, 1968.

_____. "Political Aspects of Mobility in
China's Urban Development." _American Political
Science Review_ 60 (1966):899-912.

Lindblom, Charles E. "The Science of 'Muddling
Through.'" _Public Administration Review_ 19,
no. 2 (1959):79-88.

Lowenthal, Richard. "Development vs. Utopia in
Communist Policy." _Change in Communist Systems_.
Edited by Chalmers Johnson. Stanford: Stan-
ford University Press, 1970.

"The Mao-Liu Controversy Over Rural Public Health."
Current Scene 7, no. 12 (1969):1-18.

"Mao's Revolution in Public Health." Current Scene
6, no. 7 (1968):1-10.

Mao Tse-tung. "Directive on Public Health." Chairman Mao Talks to the People. Edited by Stuart
Schram. New York: Random House, 1974.

Oksenberg, Michel. "The Chinese Policy Process and
the Public Health Issue: An Arena Approach."
Studies in Comparative Communism 7, no. 4
(1974):375-408.

_____. "Getting Ahead and Along in Communist
China: The Ladder of Success on the Eve of the
Cultural Revolution." Party Leadership and
Revolutionary Power in China. Edited by John
Wilson Lewis. London: Cambridge University
Press, 1970.

_____. "Occupational Groups in Chinese Society
and the Cultural Revolution." The Cultural
Revolution: 1967 in Review. Michigan Papers
in Chinese Studies, no. 2. Ann Arbor: Center
for Chinese Studies, University of Michigan,
1968.

_____. "Policy Making Under Mao, 1949-68: An
Overview." China: Management of a Revolution-
ary Society. Edited by John M. H. Lindbeck.
Seattle: University of Washington Press, 1971.

Orleans, Leo A. "China's Population: Can the Contradictions be Resolved?" China: A Reassess-
ment of the Economy. Washington, D.C.: Joint
Economic Committee, 1975.

_____. "China's Science and Technology: Con-
tinuity and Innovation." People's Republic
of China: An Economic Assessment. Washington,
D.C.: Joint Economic Committee, 1972.

_____. "Health Policies and Services in China,
1974." Prepared for Subcommittee on Health,
Committee on Labor and Public Welfare, United
States Senate, March 1974.

_____. "Science in China and U.S.-China Sci-
entific Exchanges: Assessment and Prospects."
Committee on Science and Technology, U.S. House
of Representatives, November 1976.

Penfield, Wilder. "Oriental Renaissance in Education and Medicine." Science 141, no. 3586
(1963):1153-1161.

Pruitt, Dean. "Definition of the Situation as a
Determinant of International Action." Inter-
national Behavior: A Social Psychological
Analysis. Edited by Herbert Kelman. New York:
Holt, Rinehart and Winston, 1966.

"Public Health Developments: Continued Focus on the
Farms." Current Scene 7, no. 24 (1969):2-12.

Russell, Maud. "China 1963: Food, Medicine,
People's Communes." Far East Reporter, n.d.

_____. "Medicine and Public Health in the
People's Republic of China." Far East Reporter,
n.d.

Salaff, Janet. "Physician Heal Thyself." Far
Eastern Economic Review 60 (1968):291-293.

Sidel, Ruth. "The Role of Revolutionary Optimism in
the Treatment of Mental Illness in the People's
Republic of China." American Journal of Orthopsychiatry 43, no. 5 (1973):732-736.

Sidel, Victor W., and Sidel, Ruth. "The Delivery of
Medical Care in China." Scientific American
230, no. 4 (1974):19-27.

Sidel, Victor W. "The Barefoot Doctors of the
People's Republic of China." New England Journal of Medicine 286 (1972):1292-1300.

_____. "Feldshers and Feldsherism." New England
Journal of Medicine 278 (1968):935-937.

_____. "The Health Workers of the Fengsheng
Neighborhood of Peking." American Journal of
Orthopsychiatry 43, no. 5 (1973):737-743.

_____. "Medical Education in the People's
Republic of China." The New Physician (1972):
284-291.

_____. "Medical Personnel and Their Training."
Medicine and Public Health in the People's
Republic of China. Edited by Joseph R. Quinn.
Washington, D.C.: National Institutes of
Health, 1972.

_____. "Some Observations on the Health Services in the People's Republic of China." _International Journal of Health Services_ 2, no. 3 (1972):385-395.

Sieh, Marie. "Medicine in China: Wealth for the State." _Current Scene_ 3, no. 6 (1964):1-15.

Skinner, G. William. "Marketing and Social Structure in Rural China, Part III." _Journal of Asian Studies_ 24, no. 3 (1965):363-399.

Skinner, G. William, and Winckler, Edwin A. "Compliance Succession in Rural Communist China: A Cyclical Theory." _A Sociological Reader on Complex Organizations_. Edited by Amitai Etzioni. New York: Holt, Rinehart, and Winston, 1969.

Suttmeier, Richard P. "The Academy of Medical Sciences." _Medicine and Public Health in the People's Republic of China_. Edited by Joseph R. Quinn. Washington, D.C.: National Institutes of Health, 1972.

_____. "Party Views of Science: The Record from the First Decade." _China Quarterly_, no. 44 (1970):146-168.

_____. "Science Policy Shifts, Organizational Change and China's Development." _China Quarterly_, no. 62 (1975):207-241.

Vogel, Ezra F. "Organization of Health Services." _Public Health in the People's Republic of China_. Edited by Myron E. Wegman, Tsung-yi Lin, and Elizabeth F. Purcell. New York: The Josiah Macy, Jr. Foundation, 1973.

White, Lynn T. "Workers' Politics in Shanghai." _Journal of Asian Studies_ 36, no. 1 (1976):99-116.

Worth, Robert M. "Health Trends in China Since the Great Leap Forward." _American Journal of Hygiene_ 78 (1963):349-357.

_____. "Institution Building in the People's Republic of China: The Rural Health Centre." Mimeographed.

BOOKS

Aird, John S. Population Estimates for the Provinces
     of the People's Republic of China: 1953 to
     1974. Washington, D.C.: Department of Com-
     merce, 1974.

Akhtar, Shahid. Health Care in the People's Repub-
     lic of China: A Bibliography with Abstracts.
     Ottawa: International Development Research
     Centre, 1975.

Allan, Ted, and Gordon, Sydney. The Scalpel, the
     Sword: The Story of Doctor Norman Bethune.
     New York: Monthly Review Press, 1973.

Almond, Gabriel A., and Powell, G. Bingham. Compar-
     ative Politics: A Developmental Approach.
     Boston: Little, Brown and Company, 1966.

Anderson, James E. Public Policy-Making. New York:
     Praeger, 1975.

The Asia Society. Science and Medicine in the
     People's Republic of China. New York: Asia
     Society, 1972.

Baker, Timothy D., and Perlman, Mark. Health Man-
     power in a Developing Economy: Taiwan, A Case
     Study in Planning. Baltimore: Johns Hopkins
     Press, 1967.

Barnett, A. Doak. Cadres, Bureaucracy, and Politi-
     cal Power in Communist China. New York:
     Columbia University Press, 1967.

_____. Chinese Communist Politics in Action.
     Seattle: University of Washington Press, 1969.

Belden, Jack. China Shakes the World. New York:
     Monthly Review Press, 1970.

Bennett, Gordon A., and Montaperto, Ronald N. Red
     Guard: The Political Biography of Dai Hsiao-ai.
     Garden City: Doubleday and Company, Inc., 1972.

Bentley, Arthur. The Process of Government. Bloom-
     ington: Principia Press, 1935.

Blau, Peter, and Scott, R. W. Formal Organizations.
     San Francisco: Chandler Publishing Company,
     1962.

Bowers, John Z. Western Medicine in a Chinese Palace: Peking Union Medical College, 1917-1951. New York: The Josiah Macy, Jr. Foundation, 1972.

Bryant, John. Health and the Developing World. Ithaca: Cornell University Press, 1969.

Chandra-sekhar, Sripati. Red China: An Asian View. New York: Praeger, 1961.

Chang, Parris H. Power and Policy in China. University Park: Pennsylvania State University Press, 1975.

Chen, C. S., and Ridley, Charles P. Rural People's Communes in Lien-chiang. Stanford: Hoover Institution Press, 1969.

Ch'ên, Jerome. Mao and the Chinese Revolution. London: Oxford University Press, 1965.

_____. Mao. Englewood Cliffs, N.J.: Prentice Hall, Inc., 1969.

Chen Nai-ruenn. Chinese Economic Statistics: A Handbook for Mainland China. Chicago: Aldine, 1967.

Croizier, Ralph C., ed. China's Cultural Legacy and Communism. New York: Praeger, 1970.

_____. Traditional Medicine and Modern China: Science, Nationalism, and the Tensions of Cultural Change. Cambridge: Harvard University Press, 1968.

Donnithorne, Audrey. China's Economic System. New York: Praeger, 1967.

Eckstein, Harry. The English Health Service: Its Origins, Structure, and Achievements. Cambridge: Harvard University Press, 1958.

_____. Pressure Group Politics: The Case of the British Medical Association. Stanford: Stanford University Press, 1960.

Ehrenreich, Barbara, and Ehrenreich, John. The American Health Empire: Power, Profits and Politics. New York: Vintage, 1971.

293

Ferguson, Mary E. China Medical Board and Peking
    Union Medical College: A Chronicle of Fruitful
    Collaboration, 1914-1951. New York: China
    Medical Board, 1970.

Field, Mark G. Soviet Socialized Medicine. New
    York: Free Press, 1967.

Friedrich, Carl J., and Brzezinski, Zbigniew K.
    Totalitarian Dictatorship and Autocracy. New
    York: Praeger, 1972.

Fry, John. Medicine in Three Countries. New York:
    American Elsevier Publishing Company, 1970.

Gamble, Sidney D. Ting Hsien: A North China Rural
    Community. Stanford: Stanford University
    Press, 1968.

Harris, Seymour. The Economics of American Medicine.
    New York: McMillan and Company, 1964.

Ho Ping-ti. Studies on the Population of China,
    1368-1953. Cambridge: Harvard University
    Press, 1967.

Hoover Institution. Directory of Selected Scientific
    Institutions in Mainland China. Stanford:
    Hoover Institution Press, 1970.

Horn, Joshua S. Away with all Pests: An English
    Surgeon in People's China: 1954-1969. New
    York: Monthly Review Press, 1969.

Hunter, Neale. Shanghai Journal: An Eyewitness
    Account of the Cultural Revolution. New York:
    Praeger, 1969.

Jen-min Shou-ts'e [People's handbook]. Peking:
    Ta-kung She, 1959, 1960, 1963, 1964.

Kessen, William, ed. Childhood in China. New Haven:
    Yale University Press, 1975.

King, Maurice. Medical Care in Developing Countries.
    London: Oxford University Press, 1966.

Klein, Donald W., and Clark, Anne B. Biographic
    Dictionary of Chinese Communism. Cambridge:
    Harvard University Press, 1971.

294

Lampton, David M. Health, Conflict, and the Chinese Political System. Michigan Papers in Chinese Studies, no. 18. Ann Arbor: Center for Chinese Studies, University of Michigan, 1974.

Lewis, John Wilson, ed. The City in Communist China. Stanford: Stanford University Press, 1971.

_____. Leadership in Communist China. Ithaca: Cornell University Press, 1963.

Lieberthal, Kenneth. A Research Guide to Central Party and Government Meetings in China, 1949-1975. White Plains, New York: International Arts and Sciences Press, Inc., 1976.

Lindbeck, John M. H., ed. China: Management of a Revolutionary Society. Seattle: University of Washington Press, 1971.

Lindblom, Charles E. The Intelligence of Democracy. New York: The Free Press, 1965.

Lu Hsun. Selected Stories of Lu Hsun. Peking: Foreign Languages Press, 1972.

MacFarquhar, Roderick. The Hundred Flowers. London: Stevens and Sons, Ltd., 1960.

_____. The Origins of the Cultural Revolution: Contradictions Among the People, 1956-1957. New York: Columbia University Press, 1974.

Mallory, Walter H. China: Land of Famine. New York: American Geographical Society, 1926.

Mao Tse-tung. Mao Tse-tung Chi [The collected writings of Mao Tse-tung]. Tokyo: Ho Tien Wu Szu, 1971.

_____. Mao Tse-tung Hsüan-chi [The selected works of Mao Tse-tung]. Peking: People's Publishing House, 1961.

_____. Mao Tse-tung Ssu-hsiang Wan-sui [Long live the thought of Mao Tse-tung]. Peking, 1967.

_____. Mao Tse-tung Ssu-hsiang Wan-sui [Long live the thought of Mao Tse-tung]. Peking, 1969.

295

_____. Poems of Mao Tse-tung. Hong Kong. Eastern Horizon Press, 1966.

_____. Selected Readings from the Works of Mao Tse-tung. Peking: Foreign Languages Press, 1971.

_____. Ten More Poems of Mao Tse-tung. Hong Kong: Eastern Horizon Press, 1967.

Munro, Donald J. The Concept of Man in Early China. Stanford: Stanford University Press, 1969.

Myrdal, Gunnar. Asian Drama: An Inquiry Into the Poverty of Nations. New York: Vintage Books, 1972.

Oksenberg, Michel, ed. China's Developmental Experience. New York: Praeger, 1973.

Orleans, Leo A. Every Fifth Child: The Population of China. Stanford: Stanford University Press, 1972.

_____. Professional Manpower and Education in Communist China. Washington, D.C.: National Science Foundation, 1961.

Ridley, Charles P. China's Scientific Policies: Implications for International Cooperation. Stanford: Hoover Institution, 1976.

Robinson, Thomas W., ed. The Cultural Revolution in China. Berkeley: University of California Press, 1971.

Roy, David T. Kuo Mo-jo: The Early Years. Cambridge: Harvard University Press, 1971.

Schram, Stuart, ed. Chairman Mao Talks to the People: Talks and Letters, 1956-1971. New York: Pantheon, 1974.

Schurmann, Franz. Ideology and Organization in Communist China. Berkeley: University of California Press, 1966.

Selden, Mark. The Yenan Way in Revolutionary China. Cambridge: Harvard University Press, 1972.

Selznick, Philip. TVA and the Grass Roots: A Study in the Sociology of Formal Organization.

Berkeley: University of California Press, 1949.

Sidel, Ruth. Women and Child Care in China. New York: Hill and Wang, 1972.

Sidel, Victor W., and Sidel, Ruth. Serve the People: Observations on Medicine in the People's Republic of China. New York: The Josiah Macy, Jr. Foundation, 1973.

Skilling, H. Gordon, and Griffiths, Franklyn, eds. Interest Groups in Soviet Politics. Princeton: Princeton University Press, 1971.

Smedley, Agnes. The Great Road: The Life and Times of Chu Teh. New York: Monthly Review Press, 1956.

Spence, Jonathan. To Change China. Boston: Little, Brown and Company, 1969.

Steslicke, William E. Doctors in Politics: The Political Life of the Japan Medical Association. New York: Praeger, 1973.

Swartz, Marc J. Local Level Politics. Chicago: Aldine, 1968.

Ten Great Years: Statistics of the Economic and Cultural Achievements of the People's Republic of China. Peking: Foreign Languages Press, 1960.

Townsend, James R. Politics in China. Boston: Little,Brown and Company, 1974.

Truman, David B. The Governmental Process: Political Interests and Public Opinion. New York: Alfred A. Knopf, 1951.

Tunley, Roul. The American Health Scandal. New York: Harper and Row, 1966.

Union Research Institute. The Case of P'eng Teh-huai: 1959-1968. Hong Kong: Union Press, 1968.

_____. CCP Documents of the Great Proletarian Cultural Revolution: 1966-1967. Hong Kong: Union Press, 1968.

_____. Communist China, 1955. Hong Kong: Union Press, 1956.

_____. Documents of Chinese Communist Party Central Committee: September 1956-April 1969. Hong Kong: Union Press, 1971.

_____. Who's Who in Communist China. Hong Kong: Union Press, 1970.

Veith, Ilza. The Yellow Emperor's Classic of Internal Medicine. Berkeley: University of California Press, 1970.

Vogel, Ezra F. Canton Under Communism: Programs and Politics in a Provincial Capital, 1949-1968. Cambridge: Harvard University Press, 1969.

Vollmer, Howard, and Mills, Donald. Professionalism. New York: Prentice-Hall, 1966.

Ward, Richard A. The Economics of Health Resources. Menlo Park: Addison-Wesley Publishing Company, 1975.

Weber, Max. The Theory of Social and Economic Organization. New York: The Free Press, 1969.

Wegman, Myron E., Lin Tsung-yi, and Purcell, Elizabeth F., eds. Public Health in the People's Republic of China. New York: The Josiah Macy, Jr. Foundation, 1973.

Weinerman, E. R. Social Medicine in Eastern Europe. Cambridge: Harvard University Press, 1969.

Wheelwright, E. L., and McFarlane, Bruce. The Chinese Road to Socialism. New York: Monthly Review Press, 1970.

Wilensky, Harold L. The Welfare State and Equality. Berkeley: University of California Press, 1975.

INTERVIEWS

Lampton, David M. Interviews with Medical Personnel, Hong Kong: 1972-1973. Each person was assigned an alphabetical letter in File 21.

Oksenberg, Michel. Interviews with Finance Official, 1965.

Rifkin, Susan B. Interviews with Traditional Chinese
     Physicians, Hong Kong: 1972-1973.

Vogel, Ezra, F. Interviews with Medical Personnel,
     Hong Kong: 1963.

PERIODICALS

Ch'ang-chiang Jih-pao [Yangtze river daily], Hankow,
     1950-1956.

Chieh-fang Jih-pao [Liberation daily], Shanghai,
     1953.

Chien-k'ang Pao [Health bulletin], Peking: Ministry
     of Public Health, 1956-1957.

China News Summary, Hong Kong: Regional Information
     Service.

China's Medicine, Peking: Chinese Medical Associa-
     tion, 1966-1968.

Ch'ing-tao Jih-pao [Tsingtao daily], Tsingtao, 1952
     and 1955.

Ch'üan-wu-ti [Invincible], Peking: Chien-k'ang Pao
     Yenan Commune, 1967.

Chung-hua I-hsüeh Tsa-chih [Chinese medical journal],
     Peking: Chinese Medical Association, 1948-1966
     and 1973-.

Chung-kuo Hsin-wen [China news], Peking, 1958-1959,
     1962-1963, and 1969.

Current Background, Hong Kong: United States Con-
     sulate General, 1951-.

Foreign Broadcast Information Service, Daily Report:
     People's Republic of China, Washington, D.C.:
     U.S. Department of Commerce, 1972-.

Fu-kien Jih-pao [Fukien daily], Foochow, 1952.

Hsiang-kang Shih-pao [Hong Kong times], Hong Kong,
     1958.

Hsin Kuan-ch'a Pan-yüeh-k'an [The new investigation
     semi-monthly], 1959.

299

Hsin Hua [New China news agency], Peking, 1949-1973.

Hsin Min Wan-pao [New people evening paper],
    Shanghai, 1965.

Hsin-wen Jih-pao [Daily news], Shanghai, 1953.

Hung Ch'i [Red flag], Peking, 1958-.

Jen-min Jih-pao [People's daily], Peking, 1949-.

K'o-hsüeh Kuo-pao [Scientific monthly], Peking, 1962.

Kuang-chou Jih-pao [Canton daily], Canton, 1953 and
    1958.

Kuang-ming Jih-pao [Bright daily], Peking, 1954-1963.

Kuang-si Jih-pao [Kwangsi daily], Kwangsi, 1956.

Ku-lin Jih-pao [Kirin daily], Kirin, 1956.

Lu-ta Jih-pao [Luta daily], Luta, 1956-1957.

Nan-ching Jih-pao [Nanking daily], Nanking, 1956.

Nan-fang Jih-pao [Southern daily], Canton, 1953-1965.

Pei-ching Jih-pao [Peking daily], Peking, 1957 and
    1962.

Pei-ching Kung-she [Peking commune], Peking, 1967.

Pei-ching Wan-pao [Peking evening paper], Peking,
    1962.

Peking Review, Peking, 1958-.

Selections From China Mainland Magazines, Hong Kong:
    U.S. Consulate General, 1960-.

Selections From China Mainland Magazines-Supplement,
    Hong Kong: U.S. Consulate General, 1967-.

Shan-si Jih-pao [Shansi daily], Shansi, 1955 and
    1957.

Sheng-yang Jih-pao [Shengyang daily], Shengyang,
    1955-1957.

South China Morning Post, Hong Kong, 1965 and 1972-
    1973.

Survey of China Mainland Press, Hong Kong: U.S.
      Consulate General, 1950-.

Survey of China Mainland Press-Supplement, Hong Kong:
      U.S. Consulate General, 1966-.

Ta-kung Pao [Impartial daily], Peking, 1956.

Ta-kung Pao [Impartial daily], Tientsin, 1951 and
      1956.

T'ien-ching Jih-pao [Tientsin daily], 1951, 1953,
      and 1956.